Nursing

Scope and Standards of Practice

3rd Edition

AMERICAN NURSES
ASSOCIATION

American Nurses Association
Silver Spring, Maryland 2015

The American Nurses Association (ANA) is a national professional association. This ANA publication, *Nursing: Scope and Standards of Practice, Third Edition*, reflects the thinking of the nursing profession on various issues and should be reviewed in conjunction with state board of nursing policies and practices. State law, rules, and regulations govern the practice of nursing, while *Nursing: Scope and Standards of Practice, Third Edition*, guides nurses in the application of their professional knowledge, skills, and responsibilities.

American Nurses Association
8515 Georgia Avenue, Suite 400
Silver Spring, MD 20910-3492
1-800-274-4ANA
http://www.Nursingworld.org

Cataloging-in-Publication Data on file with the Library of Congress

ISBN-13: 978-1-55810-619-2   SAN: 851-3481   03/2016R

First printing: July 2015.
Second printing: November 2015.
Third printing: March 2016.

Contents

Contributors

Nursing: Scope and Standards of Practice, Third Edition, is the product of extensive thought work by many registered nurses and a three-step review process. This document originated from the decisions garnered during a significant number of telephone conference calls and electronic mail communications of the diverse workgroup members and an intensive two-day in person weekend meeting. The first review process, a 30-day public comment period, followed. All workgroup members reviewed every comment, resulting in further workgroup refinements of the draft document. The official American Nurses Association (ANA) review process included evaluation by the Committee on Nursing Practice Standards and final review and approval by the ANA Board of Directors in June 2015. The list of endorsing organizations that completes this section reflects the broad acceptance of this resource within the profession.

Nursing Scope and Standards Workgroup, 2014–2015

Elizabeth Thomas, MEd, RN, NCSN, FNASN, Chairperson

Chad Allen, RN

Sheri-Lynne Almeida, DrPH, MSN, MED, RN, CEN, FAEN

Carolyn Baird, DNP, MBA, RN-BC, CARN-AP, CCDPD, FIAAN

Nancy Barr, MSN, RN

Patricia Bartzak, DNP, RN, CMSRN

Mavis Bechtle, MSN, RN

Jennifer Bellot, PhD, MHSE, RN, CNE

Tom Blodgett, PhD, MSN, GCNS, RN-BC

Patricia Bowe, MS, BSN, RN

Katreena Collette-Merrill, PhD, RN

Kahlil Demonbreun, DNP, RNC-OB, WHNP-BC, ANP-BC

Sheila Eason, MS, BSN, RN, CNOR

Tim Fish, DNP, MBA, RN, CENP

Matthew French-Bravo, MSN, RN

Heather Healy, MS, APRN, FNP-BC, NEA-BC

Susan Howard, MSN, RN-BC

Brenda Hutchins, DNP, ANP-BC, GNP-BC

Lorinda Inman, MSN, RN, FRE

Donna Konradi, PhD, RN, CNE

Mary Ann Lavin, ScD, APRN, ANP-BC, FNI, FAAN

Carla Mariano, EdD, RN, AHN-BC, FAAIM

Lucy Marion, PhD, RN, FAANP, FAAN

Deborah Maust Martin, DNP, MBA, RN, NE-BC, FACHE

Cindy McCullough, MSN, CMSRN, AGCNS-BC

Kris A. McLoughlin, DNP; APRN; PMH-CNS, BC; CADC-II, FAAN

Joyce Morris, MSN, RN-BC

Sandra J. Fulton Picot, PhD, RN, CLNC, FGSA, FAAN

Deborah Poling, PhD, RN, FNP-BC, CNE

Lori L. Profata, DNP, RN, NE-BC

Karen Rea-Williams, MS, FNP

ShyRhonda Roy, MSN, RN

Debbie Ruiz, RN

Kathryn Schroeter, PhD, RN, CNE, CNOR

Melida Shepard, RN, BSN, CPHQ

Suzanne Sikes-Thurman, BA, BSN, RN

Janice Smolowitz, EdD, DNP, RN, ANP-BC

Lynn Tomascik, MSN, RN

Linda Wagner, MA, RN, NE-BC

Acknowledgment of Special Contribution

Marilyn (Marty) Douglas, PhD, RN, FAAN

ANA Committee on Nursing Practice Standards

Richard Henker, PhD, RN, CRNA, FAAN: co- chair 03/2014–12/2015

Tresha (Terry) L. Lucas, MSN, RN: co- chair 07/2011–12/2014

Danette Culver, MSN, APRN, ACNS-BC, CCRN

Deborah Finnell, DNS, PMHNP-BC, CARN-AP, FAAN

Renee Gecsedi, MS, RN

Deedra Harrington, DNP, MSN, APRN, ACNP-BC

Maria Jurlano, MS, BSN, RN, NEA-BC, CCRN

Carla A. B. Lee, PhD, APRN-BC, CNAA, FAAN, FIBA

Verna Sitzer, PhD, RN, CNS

ANA Staff, 2014-2015

Carol J. Bickford, PhD, RN-BC, CPHIMS, FAAN – Content editor

Mary Jo Assi, DNP, RN, FNP-BC, NEA-BC

Maureen E. Cones, Esq. – Legal Counsel

Eric Wurzbacher, BA – Project editor

Yvonne Humes, MSA – Project assistant

About the American Nurses Association

The American Nurses Association (ANA) is the only full-service professional organization representing the interests of the nation's 3.4 million registered nurses through its constituent member nurses associations and its organizational affiliates. ANA advances the nursing profession by fostering high standards of nursing practice, promoting the rights of nurses in the workplace, projecting a positive and realistic view of nursing, and by lobbying the Congress and regulatory agencies on healthcare issues affecting nurses and the public.

About Nursesbooks.org, The Publishing Program of ANA

Nursesbooks.org publishes books on ANA core issues and programs, including ethics, leadership, quality, specialty practice, advanced practice, and the profession's enduring legacy. Best known for the Essential documents of the profession on nursing ethics, scope and standards of practice, and social policy, Nursesbooks.org is the publisher for the professional, career-oriented nurse, reaching and serving nurse educators, administrators, managers, and researchers as well as staff nurses in the course of their professional development.

Overview of the Content

Essential Documents of Professional Nursing

Registered nurses practicing in the United States have two contemporary professional resources that inform their thinking and decision-making and guide their practice. First, the *Code of Ethics for Nurses with Interpretive Statements* (American Nurses Association, 2015) lists the nine succinct provisions and accompanying interpretive statements that establish the ethical framework for registered nurses' practice across all roles, levels, and settings. Secondly, the 2015 *Nursing: Scope and Standards of Practice, Third Edition*, outlines the expectations of professional nursing practice. The scope of practice statement presents the framework and context of nursing practice and accompanies the standards of professional nursing practice and their associated competencies that identify the evidence of the standard of care.

Additional Content

For a better appreciation of the history, content, and context related to *Nursing: Scope and Standards of Practice, Third Edition*, readers will find the additional content of the six appendices useful:

- Appendix A. *Nursing: Scope and Standards of Practice, Second Edition* (2010)

- Appendix B. *Nursing's Social Policy Statement: The Essence of the Profession* (2010)

- Appendix C. ANA Position Statement : *Professional Role Competence* (2014)

- Appendix D. The Development of Essential Nursing Documents and Professional Nursing

- Appendix E. List of Selected Nurse Theorists

- Appendix F. Culturally Congruent Practice Resources

Audience for This Publication

Registered nurses in every clinical and functional role and setting constitute the primary audience of this professional resource. Students, interprofessional colleagues, agencies, and organizations also will find this an invaluable reference. Legislators, regulators, legal counsel, and the judiciary will also want to examine this content. In addition, the individuals, families, groups, communities, and populations using nursing and healthcare services can use this document to better understand what constitutes the profession of nursing and how registered nurses and advanced practice registered nurses lead within today's healthcare environment.

Scope of Nursing Practice

Definition of Nursing

The following contemporary definition of nursing has been slightly modified from that published in the 2003 *Nursing's Social Policy Statement, Second Edition,* and included in the 2004 and 2010 editions of *Nursing: Scope and Standards of Practice,* with the inclusion of "facilitation of healing" and "groups":

> *Nursing is the protection, promotion, and optimization of health and abilities, prevention of illness and injury, facilitation of healing, alleviation of suffering through the diagnosis and treatment of human response, and advocacy in the care of individuals, families, groups, communities, and populations.*

This definition serves as the foundation for the following expanded descriptions of the Scope of Nursing Practice and the Standards of Professional Nursing Practice.

Professional Nursing's Scope and Standards of Practice

A professional organization has a responsibility to its members and to the public it serves to develop the scope and standards of practice for its profession. The American Nurses Association (ANA), the professional organization for all registered nurses, has long assumed the responsibility for developing and maintaining the scope of practice statement and standards that apply to the practice of all professional nurses and also serve as a template for evaluation of nursing specialty practice. Both the scope and standards do, however, belong to the profession and thus require broad input into their development and revision. *Nursing: Scope and Standards of Practice, Third Edition* describes a competent level of nursing practice and professional performance common to all registered nurses.

Description of the Scope of Nursing Practice

The Scope of Nursing Practice describes the "who," "what," "where," "when," "why," and "how" of nursing practice. Each of these questions must be answered to provide a complete picture of the dynamic and complex practice of nursing and its evolving boundaries and membership. The definition of nursing provides a succinct characterization of the "what" of nursing. Registered nurses and advanced practice registered nurses comprise the "who" constituency and have been educated, titled, and maintain active licensure to practice nursing. Nursing occurs "when"ever there is a need for nursing knowledge, wisdom, caring, leadership, practice, or education, anytime, anywhere. Nursing occurs in any environment "where" there is a healthcare consumer in need of care, information, or advocacy. The "how" of nursing practice is defined as the ways, means, methods, and manners that nurses use to practice professionally. The "why" is characterized as nursing's response to the changing needs of society to achieve positive healthcare consumer outcomes in keeping with nursing's social contract with an obligation to society. The depth and breadth in which individual registered nurses and advanced practice registered nurses engage in the total scope of nursing practice is dependent on their education, experience, role, and the population served.

These definitions are provided to promote clarity and understanding for all readers:

Healthcare consumers are the patients, persons, clients, families, groups, communities, or populations who are the focus of attention and to whom the registered nurse is providing services as sanctioned by the state regulatory bodies. This more global term is intended to reflect a proactive focus on health and wellness care, rather than a reactive perspective to disease and illness.

Registered nurses (RNs) are individuals who are educationally prepared and licensed by a state, commonwealth, territory, government, or regulatory body to practice as a registered nurse. "Nurse" and "professional nurse" are synonyms for a registered nurse in this document.

Graduate-level prepared registered nurses are registered nurses prepared at the master's or doctoral educational level; have advanced knowledge, skills, abilities, and judgment; function in an advanced level as designated by elements of the nurse's position; and are not required to have additional regulatory oversight.

Advanced practice registered nurses (APRNs) are registered nurses:

- Who have completed an accredited graduate-level education program preparing the nurse for one of the four recognized APRN roles [certified registered nurse anesthetist (CRNA), certified nurse midwife (CNM), clinical nurse specialist (CNS), or certified nurse practitioner (CNP)];

- Who have passed a national certification examination that measures APRN-, role-, and population-focused competencies and maintain continued competence as evidenced by recertification in the role and population through the national certification program;

- Who have acquired advanced clinical knowledge and skills preparing the nurse to provide direct care to patients, as well as a component of indirect care; however, the defining factor for all APRNs is that a significant component of the education and practice focuses on direct care of individuals;

- Whose practices build on the competencies of registered nurses (RNs) by demonstrating a greater depth and breadth of knowledge, a greater synthesis of data, increased complexity of skills and interventions, and greater role autonomy;

- Who are educationally prepared to assume responsibility and accountability for health promotion and/or maintenance as well as the assessment, diagnosis, and management of patient problems, which includes the use and prescription of pharmacologic and non-pharmacologic interventions;

- Who have clinical experience of sufficient depth and breadth to reflect the intended license; and

- Who have obtained a license to practice as an APRN in one of the four APRN roles: certified registered nurse anesthetist (CRNA), certified nurse midwife (CNM), clinical nurse specialist (CNS), or certified nurse practitioner (CNP) (APRN Joint Dialogue Group, 2008).

Development and Function of the Standards of Professional Nursing Practice

The Scope of Practice Statement is accompanied by the Standards of Professional Nursing Practice. The standards are authoritative statements of the duties that all registered nurses, regardless of role, population, or specialty, are expected to perform competently. The standards published herein may serve as evidence of the standard of care, with the understanding that application of the standards depends on context. The standards are subject to change with the dynamics of the nursing profession, as new patterns of professional practice are developed and accepted by the nursing profession and the public. In addition, specific conditions and clinical circumstances may also affect the application of the standards at a given time, e.g., during a natural disaster or epidemic. As with the scope of practice statement, the standards are subject to formal, periodic review, and revision.

The Standards of Professional Nursing Practice consist of the Standards of Practice and the Standards of Professional Performance.

Standards of Practice

The Standards of Practice describe a competent level of nursing care as demonstrated by the critical thinking model known as the nursing process. The nursing process includes the components of assessment, diagnosis, outcomes identification, planning, implementation, and evaluation. Accordingly, the nursing process encompasses significant actions taken by registered nurses and forms the foundation of the nurse's decision-making.

Standard 1. Assessment

The registered nurse collects pertinent data and information relative to the healthcare consumer's health or the situation.

Standard 2. Diagnosis

The registered nurse analyzes the assessment data to determine actual or potential diagnoses, problems, and issues.

Standard 3. Outcomes Identification

The registered nurse identifies expected outcomes for a plan individualized to the healthcare consumer or the situation.

Standard 4. Planning

The registered nurse develops a plan that prescribes strategies to attain expected, measurable outcomes.

Standard 5. Implementation

The registered nurse implements the identified plan.

Standard 5A. Coordination of Care

The registered nurse coordinates care delivery.

Standard 5B. Health Teaching and Health Promotion

The registered nurse employs strategies to promote health and a safe environment.

Standard 6. Evaluation

The registered nurse evaluates progress toward attainment of goals and outcomes.

Standards of Professional Performance

The Standards of Professional Performance describe a competent level of behavior in the professional role, including activities related to ethics, culturally congruent practice, communication, collaboration, leadership, education, evidence-based practice and research, quality of practice, professional practice evaluation, resource utilization, and environmental health. All registered nurses are expected to engage in professional role activities, including leadership, appropriate to their education and position. Registered nurses are accountable for their professional actions to themselves, their healthcare consumers, their peers, and ultimately to society.

Standard 7. Ethics

The registered nurse practices ethically.

Standard 8. Culturally Congruent Practice

The registered nurse practices in a manner that is congruent with cultural diversity and inclusion principles.

Standard 9. Communication

The registered nurse communicates effectively in all areas of practice.

Standard 10. Collaboration

The registered nurse collaborates with healthcare consumer and other key stakeholders in the conduct of nursing practice.

Standard 11. Leadership

The registered nurse leads within the professional practice setting and the profession.

Standard 12. Education

The registered nurse seeks knowledge and competence that reflects current nursing practice and promotes futuristic thinking.

Standard 13. Evidence-based Practice and Research
The registered nurse integrates evidence and research findings into practice.

Standard 14. Quality of Practice
The registered nurse contributes to quality nursing practice.

Standard 15. Professional Practice Evaluation
The registered nurse evaluates one's own and others' nursing practice.

Standard 16. Resource Utilization
The registered nurse utilizes appropriate resources to plan, provide, and sustain evidence-based nursing services that are safe, effective, and fiscally responsible.

Standard 17. Environmental Health
The registered nurse practices in an environmentally safe and healthy manner.

The Function of Competencies in Standards
The competencies that accompany each standard may be evidence of demonstrated compliance with the corresponding standard. The list of competencies is not exhaustive. Whether a particular standard or competency applies depends upon the circumstances. For example, a nurse providing treatment to an unconscious, critical healthcare consumer who presented to the hospital by ambulance without family has a duty to collect comprehensive data pertinent to the healthcare consumer's health (Standard 1. Assessment). However, under the attendant circumstances, that nurse may not be expected "to assess family dynamics and impact on the healthcare consumer's health and wellness" (one of Starndard 1's competencies). In the same instance, Standard 5B. Health Teaching and Health Promotion might not apply at all.

Integrating the Art and Science of Nursing

Nursing is a learned profession built on a core body of knowledge that reflects its dual components of art and science. Nursing requires judgment and skill based on principles of the biological, physical, behavioral, and social sciences. Registered nurses employ critical thinking to integrate objective data with knowledge gained from an assessment of the subjective experiences of healthcare consumers. Registered nurses use critical thinking to apply the best available evidence and research data to diagnosis and treatment decisions. Nurses continually evaluate quality and effectiveness of nursing practice and seek to optimize outcomes.

Nursing promotes the delivery of holistic consumer-centered care and optimal health outcomes throughout the lifespan and across the health–illness continuum within an environmental context that encompasses culture, ethics, law, politics, economics, access to healthcare resources, and competing priorities. Similarly, nursing promotes the health of communities by using advocacy for social and environmental justice, community engagement, and access to high-quality and equitable health care to maximize population health outcomes and minimize health disparities. Nursing advocates for the well-being, comfort, dignity, and humanity of all individuals, families, groups, communities, and populations. Nursing focuses on healthcare consumer and interprofessional collaboration, sharing of knowledge, scientific discovery, and social welfare.

The What and How of Nursing
What Is Nursing?

What is nursing? **Nursing is the protection, promotion, and optimization of health and abilities, prevention of illness and injury, facilitation of healing, alleviation of suffering through the diagnosis and treatment of human response, and advocacy in the care of individuals, families, groups, communities, and populations.** This succinct but very powerful definition statement (see p. 11) reflects the evolution of the profession. The integration of the art and science of nursing is described in the following detailed scope and standards of practice content.

Nursing is a learned profession built on a core body of knowledge that reflects its dual components of art and science. Nursing requires judgment and skill based on principles of the biological, physical, behavioral, and social sciences.

Tenets Characteristic of Nursing Practice

The conduct of nursing practice in all settings also can be characterized by the following tenets that are reflected in language that threads throughout the scope of practice statement and standards of practice and professional performance.

1. *Caring and health are central to the practice of the registered nurse.*

    Professional nursing promotes healing and health in a way that builds a relationship between nurse and patient (Watson, 2008, 2012). "Caring is a conscious judgment that manifests itself in concrete acts, interpersonally, verbally, and nonverbally"

(Gallagher-Lepak & Kubsch, 2009, p. 171). While caring for individuals, families, groups, and populations is the key focus of nursing, the nurse additionally promotes self-care as well as care of the environment and society (Hagerty, Lynch-Sauer, Patusky, & Bouwseman, 1993; ANA, 2015).

2. *Nursing practice is individualized.*

Nursing practice respects diversity and focuses on identifying and meeting the unique needs of the healthcare consumer or situation. *Healthcare consumer* is defined to be the patient, person, client, family, group, community, or population who is the focus of attention and to whom the registered nurse is providing services as sanctioned by the state regulatory bodies.

3. *Registered nurses use the nursing process to plan and provide individualized care for healthcare consumers.*

The nursing process is cyclical and dynamic, interpersonal and collaborative, and universally applicable. Nurses use theoretical and evidence-based knowledge of human experiences and responses to collaborate with healthcare consumers to assess, diagnose, identify outcomes, plan, implement, and evaluate care that has been individualized to achieve the best outcomes. Nursing actions are intended to produce beneficial effects, contribute to quality outcomes, and above all, "do no harm." Nurses evaluate the effectiveness of care in relation to identified outcomes and use evidence-based practice to improve care. Critical thinking underlies each step of the nursing process, problem-solving, and decision-making.

4. *Nurses coordinate care by establishing partnerships.*

The registered nurse establishes partnerships with persons, families, groups, support systems, and other providers, utilizing effective in-person and electronic communications, to reach a shared goal of delivering safe, quality health care to address the health needs of the healthcare consumer and the public. The registered nurse is responsible and accountable for communicating and advocating for the planning and care coordination focused on the healthcare consumer, families, and support systems (ANA, 2013a). Collaborative interprofessional team planning is based on recognition of each individual profession's value and contributions, mutual trust, respect, open discussion, and shared decision-making.

5. *A strong link exists between the professional work environment and the registered nurse's ability to provide quality health care and achieve optimal outcomes.*

   Professional nurses have an ethical obligation to maintain and improve healthcare practice environments conducive to the provision of quality health care (ANA, 2015). Extensive studies have demonstrated the relationship between effective nursing practice and the presence of a healthy work environment. Mounting evidence demonstrates that negative, demoralizing, and unsafe conditions in the workplace (unhealthy work environments) contribute to errors, ineffective delivery of care, workplace conflict and stress, and moral distress.

The How of Nursing

The "how" of nursing practice is defined as the ways, means, methods, processes, and manner by which the registered nurse practices professionally. The **ways** in which registered nurses practice reflect integration of the five core practice competencies of all healthcare professionals: healthcare consumer-centered practice, evidence-based practice, interprofessional collaboration, use of informatics, and continuous quality improvement (Institute of Medicine, 2003). Registered nurses recognize that using a holistic approach prevents omission of relevant data when implementing the **nursing process**. When incorporating a *healthcare consumer-centered approach*, the registered nurse collaborates with and treats all healthcare consumers with the utmost respect. The registered nurse demonstrates culturally congruent practice, always advocating that healthcare consumers have sufficient information and questions answered, enabling them to exercise their autonomy to make the final decisions regarding their preferred care.

To achieve the best healthcare consumer outcomes, the "how" requires the registered nurse to employ *evidence-based practice* as a **means** to incorporate the best available evidence, healthcare consumer preferences, provider expertise, and contextual resources in which nursing is delivered. Closely linked to the best healthcare consumer outcomes is the need for effective *interprofessional collaboration*. Thus, an essential component of the "how" of registered nursing is care coordination (ANA, 2013a), requiring effective communications by all stakeholders.

Additionally, the "how" of registered nursing practice encompasses **methods** such as communicating predictably and comprehensively using approaches such as informatics, electronic health records, and established processes to prevent errors. Methods can include situation, background, assessment, recommendation (SBAR) (The Joint Commission Enterprise, 2012) and TeamSTEPPS[R] as evidence-based methods of building teamwork and communication skills (Department of Defense 2014; Agency for Healthcare Research and Quality, n.d.).

Critical to the practice of professional nursing is ethical conduct of research to generate new knowledge and translate that knowledge to practice using theory-driven approaches (Estabrooks, Thompson, Lovely, & Hofmeyer, 2006). Finally, the "how" of registered nursing practice reflects the **manner** in which the registered nurse practices according to the *Code of Ethics for Nurses with Interpretive Statements*, standards for professional nursing practice, institutional review boards' protocols, and directives of other governing and regulatory bodies that guide the conduct of professional nursing practice.

These activities reflect nursing's long-standing commitment to its responsibilities to the society out of which it grew and continues to serve. Such a professional relationship and associated expectations and contributions toward the evolution of a health-oriented system of care were first formally articulated in the 1980 *Nursing: A Social Policy Statement.* Later editions of the social policy statement in 1995, 2003, and 2010 confirmed the importance of nurse–healthcare consumer partnerships; healthcare consumers' decision-making, accountability, and responsibility of choice; and the necessary focus on healthcare consumer-centered care and outcomes.

Nursing's Social Policy Statement: The Essence of the Profession identifies the following statements that undergird professional nursing's social contract with society (ANA, 2010b, p. 6):

- Humans manifest an essential unity of mind, body, and spirit.

- Human experience is contextually and culturally defined.

- Health and illness are human experiences. The presence of illness does not preclude health, nor does optimal health preclude illness.

- The relationship between the nurse and patient occurs within the context of the values and beliefs of the patient and nurse.

- Public policy and the healthcare delivery system influence the health and well-being of society and professional nursing.

- Individual responsibility and interprofessional involvement are essential.

Consult Appendix B, *Nursing's Social Policy Statement* for discussion of other content important to understanding the societal context related to the decision-making and conduct of professional nursing practice.

The Art of Nursing

The art of nursing is based on caring and respect for human dignity. A compassionate approach to patient care carries a mandate to provide care competently. Such competent care is provided and accomplished through both independent practice and partnerships. Collaboration may be with individuals seeking support or assistance with their healthcare needs, interprofessional colleagues, and other stakeholders.

The art of nursing embraces spirituality, healing, empathy, mutual respect, and compassion. These intangible aspects promote health. Nursing embraces healing. Healing is fostered by helping, listening, mentoring, coaching, teaching, exploring, being present, supporting, touching, intuition, service, cultural competence, tolerance, acceptance, nurturing, mutually creating, and conflict resolution.

Nursing focuses on the protection, promotion, and optimization of health and quality of life; prevention or resolution of disease, illness, or disability; facilitation of healing, alleviation of suffering; and transition to a dignified and peaceful death. Nursing needs are identified from a holistic perspective and are met in the context of a culturally sensitive, caring, personal relationship. Nursing includes the diagnosis and treatment of human responses to actual or potential health problems. Registered nurses employ practices that are promotive, supportive, and restorative in nature.

Care and Caring in Nursing Practice

The act of caring is foundational to the practice of nursing: "A great truth, the act of caring is the first step in the power to heal" (Moffitt, 2004, p. 23). Watson (2012), in her *Human Caring Science Theory*, emphasizes the personal relationship between patient and nurse; highlights the role of the nurse in defining the patient as a unique human being to be valued, respected, nurtured, understood, assisted; and stresses the importance of the connections between the nurse and patient. Human care and caring is viewed as the moral ideal of nursing consisting of human-to-human attempts to protect, enhance, and preserve humanity and human dignity, integrity, and wholeness by assisting a person to find meaning in illness, suffering, pain, and existence. Human caring helps another gain self-knowledge, self-control, self-caring, and self-healing so that a sense of inner harmony is restored regardless of the external circumstances.

Human caring is not just an emotion, concern, attitude, or benevolent desire. It involves values, knowledge, caring actions, acceptance of consequences, a will, and a commitment to care. Human caring is related to intersubjective human responses to health-illness-healing conditions; a knowledge of health-illness, environmental-personal relations, and the nurse caring process; and self-knowledge in relation to both strengths and limitations. Human caring follows a process consisting of antecedents, attributes, and outcomes of caring, which go on to affect future encounters of caring.

This process includes the care recipient and the nurse, both of whom are required in a human caring relationship. The nurse must possess competence, professional maturity, interpersonal sensitivity, a moral foundation that supports caring actions, and access to a setting that is conducive to caring, while the care recipient must possess a need for and openness to caring. When combined, these antecedents can produce an intimate relationship between the care recipient and the nurse in which caring can occur to improve the physical and mental well-being of the healthcare consumer and feelings of satisfaction and renewal for the nurse.

In a caring relationship, the nurse utilizes well-honed assessment skills based on insight garnered through interpersonal sensitivity to accurately identify nuances and help find meaning in the care recipient's situation. Interventions that reflect a caring consciousness may require creativity and daring, but can also be demonstrated in simple gestures of interpersonal connection, such as attentive listening, touching, and making eye contact, and sensitivity to cultural meanings associated with caring behaviors (Finfgeld-Connett, 2007).

Caring is

- Grounded in ethics, beginning with respect for the autonomy of the care recipient,

- Grounded, as a science, in nursing, but is not limited to nursing,

- An attribute that may be taught, modeled, learned, mastered,

- Capable of being measured and analyzed scientifically,

- The subject of study within caring science institutes/academies worldwide, and

- Central to relationships that lead to effective healing, cure, and/or actualization of human potential.

The caring embraced by nursing and described here does not compete with nor is it diminished by technological advances, individual or group wealth or its absence, professional or socioeconomic status or prestige or its lack, or any other parameter that attempts to categorize the place of the person in society. The act of caring, as well as the theory and science of caring, is all-inclusive:

The nursing profession has an ethical and social responsibility to both individuals and society to sustain human caring in instances where it is threatened, and to be the guardian of human caring, individually and collectively, serving as the vanguard of society's human caring needs now and in the future. If nursing does not fulfill its societal mandate for sustaining human caring, preserving human dignity and humanness in self, systems, and society, it will not be carrying out its covenant to humankind and its reason for existence as a profession. (Watson, 2012, p. 42)

Cultural Components of Care

Leininger (1988) considered care for people from a broad range of cultures and contributed to the unique body of nursing knowledge by translating and integrating transcultural precepts from the field of anthropology into nursing science. She provided nursing with a global context, specifically exposing nursing to worldly cultures and learned behaviors, beyond those encountered within a dominant culture. Transcultural literacy has deepened nursing's holistic approach by providing a framework to better understand and provide care to culturally diverse individuals, groups, and communities.

The Science of Nursing

Nurses as scientists rely on qualitative and quantitative evidence to guide policies and practices, but also as a way of identifying the nurses' impact on the health outcomes of healthcare consumers. When describing how nurses complete professional thinking and activities, the nursing process emerges as a commonly used analytical critical thinking framework.

The nursing process is conceptualized as a cyclic, iterative, and dynamic process including assessment, diagnosis, outcomes identification, planning, implementation, and evaluation. The nursing process supports evidence-based practice and relies heavily on the bidirectional feedback loops between components, as illustrated in Figure 1. The hexagon delineates the six steps of the nursing process beginning with assessment at the 12 o'clock position, followed clockwise with diagnosis, outcomes identification, planning, implementation, and evaluation. Note the iterative actions reflected with bidirectional arrows.

The Standards of Practice included in the first ring coincide with the steps of the nursing process to represent the directive nature of the standards as the professional nurse completes each component of the nursing process. Similarly, the surrounding Standards of Professional Performance identified in the outermost ring reflect how the professional nurse adheres to the Standards of Practice, completes the nursing process, and addresses other nursing practice issues and concerns.

FIGURE 1. The Nursing Process and the Standards of Professional Nusing Practice

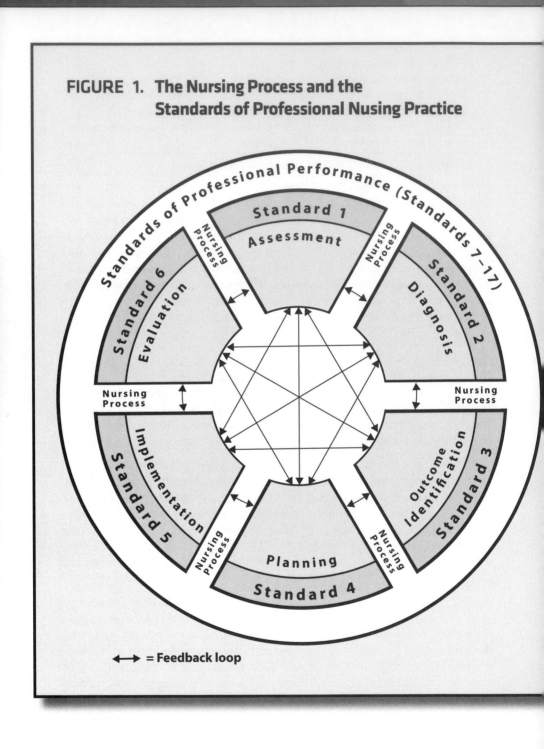

↔ = Feedback loop

The Standards of Practice

These standards describe a *competent level of nursing practice* demonstrated by the critical thinking model known as the **nursing process**; its six components correspond to these standards.

Standard	Nursing Process Component
Standard 1	Assessment
Standard 2	Diagnosis
Standard 3	Outcomes Identification
Standard 4	Planning
Standard 5	Implementation
Standard 6	Evaluation

The Standards of Professional Performance

These standards describe a *competent level of behavior in the professional role* appropriate to their education and position.

Standard	Professional Performance
Standard 7	Ethics
Standard 8	Culturally Congruent Practice
Standard 9	Communication
Standard 10	Collaboration
Standard 11	Leadership
Standard 12	Education
Standard 13	Evidence-based Practice and Research
Standard 14	Quality of Practice
Standard 15	Professional Practice Evaluation
Standard 16	Resource Utilization
Standard 17	Environmental Health

When Nursing Occurs

Nursing occurs whenever there is a need for nursing knowledge, wisdom, caring, leadership, practice, or education. The term "whenever" encompasses *anytime, anywhere, with anyone*.

Timing relates less to a point in time as measured by a clock and more to the continuum of life events that relate to past, present, and future health and responses to illness/injury. The time for nursing is: when there is need for support, guidance, healing, advocacy, nursing expertise; during life transitions, challenges, developmental and situational crises, and health maintenance; and before and during social and healthcare change. The timing of nursing refers less to when any one observation or action is made, but more to the grasping of the meaning of healthcare actions performed and outcomes attained and acting upon that meaning in a manner consistent with one's knowledge, education, and scope and standards of practice.

Nursing happens when there are *retrospective* circumstances requiring analysis and action, including root cause, risk factors, lifestyle, familial, cultural, genetic, environmental predispositions, or loss. It happens in the *present* when working with healthcare consumers within the context of their meaning applied to the diagnosis, illness, issue, problem, situation, or challenge being faced. Nursing happens when, through active and informed vigilance, nurses assess, diagnose risks, and intervene to prevent complications. Nursing happens *prospectively* when dealing with anticipatory guidance, health promotion, disease prevention, well-being, wellness, and transition.

When nursing is practiced, it is holistic and the nurse:

- Partners with the individual/family/group/community/population;

- Considers norms and values, health and illness perspectives and practices, customs, behaviors, and beliefs of the healthcare consumer; and

- Arrives at healthcare decisions that are contextualized by how the individual/family/group/community/population perceives health, the nature of the body, and its relationship to mind, emotion, energy, spirit, or environment.

Nursing Knowledge, Research, and Evidence-based Practice

Contemporary nursing practice has its historical roots in the poorhouses, the battlefields, and the industrial revolutions in 19th-century Europe and America. Initially, nurses trained in hospital-based nursing schools and were employed mainly providing private care to patients in their homes. Florence

WK 1 pg 13-19

WK 2: pp 1-11; 110

WK 3:
pg 31-45; 77; 79; 82

WK 4: pg 22-33

Hughes - EB Handbook
for Nurses

WK 5: pg 47-62

website:
- Quality Safety Education
- AHRQ Health Innovation

WK 6 pg 14; 21-31
B website

wk 7 : pg 28-30.
45-49; 75

Article :
  Mann; Gordon, Mackenzie

Reflection: Reflective
  Practice in Heath
  profession educ.

---

wk8 ∅

Nightingale provided a foundation for nursing and the basis for autonomous nursing practice as distinct from medicine. Nightingale is credited with identifying the importance of collecting empirical evidence, the underpinning of nursing's current emphasis on evidence-based practice:

> What you want are facts, not opinions.... The most important practical lesson that can be given to nurses is to teach them what to observe—how to observe—what symptoms indicate improvement—which are of none—which are the evidence of neglect—and what kind of neglect. (Nightingale, 1859, p. 105)

Although Nightingale recommended clinical nursing research in the mid-1800s, nurses did not follow her advice for over 100 years. Nursing research was able to flourish only as nurses received advanced educational preparation. In the early 1900s, nurses received advanced degrees in nursing education, and nursing research was limited to studies of nurses and nursing education. Case studies on nursing interventions were conducted in the 1920s and 1930s and the results published in the *American Journal of Nursing*.

In the 1950s, interest in nursing care studies began to rise. In 1952, the first issue of *Nursing Research* was published. In the 1960s, nursing studies began to explore theoretical and conceptual frameworks as a basis for practice. By the 1970s, more doctorally prepared nurses were conducting research, especially studies related to practice and the improvement of patient care. By the 1980s, there were greater numbers of qualified nurse researchers than ever before, and more computers available for collection and analysis of data. In 1985, the National Center for Nursing Research was established within the National Institutes of Health, putting nursing research into the mainstream of health research.

In the last half of the 20th century, nurse researchers (1950s) and nurse theorists (1960s and 1970s) greatly contributed to the expanding body of nursing knowledge with their studies of nursing practice and the development of nursing models and theories. Theories are patterns that guide the *thinking about, being,* and *doing* of nursing. Theories provide structure and substance to organize knowledge, guide practice, enhance the care of healthcare consumers, and guide inquiry to advance the science and practice of the profession. They must be flexible and dynamic to keep pace with the growth and changes in the discipline and the practice of nursing. The further development and expanded use of nursing theories and models continues today and is essential to the ongoing evolution of nursing. Appendix E includes a list of selected nurse theorists and their work.

Nursing, as an art and a science, reflects all the ways of knowing [e.g, empirical, ethical, personal, and aesthetic as identified by Carper (1978)], gleaned from: scientific investigations, accumulated and graded evidence, qualitative analysis, narratives, appreciative inquiry, case studies, interpersonal and cultural sensitivity, insight, sociopolitical awareness, intuition, experience, reflection, introspection, creative thinking, philosophical analyses, and spirituality. The practice of nursing is rooted in evidence-based knowledge. Evidence-based practice (EBP) is a life-long problem-solving approach that integrates the best evidence from well-designed research studies and evidence-based theories; clinical expertise and evidence from assessment of the health consumer's history and condition, as well as healthcare resources; and patient/family/group/community/population preferences and values. When evidence-based practice is delivered in a context of caring and a culture, as well as an ecosystem or environment that supports it, the best clinical decisions are made to yield positive healthcare consumer outcomes (Melnyk, Gallagher-Ford, Long, & Fineout-Overholt, 2014).

While outcomes are essential, the EBP process itself provides a framework for clinicians, educators, and nurse researchers to ponder, and then expertly construct the most relevant, patient-centered, and testable questions, which in turn yield important practice guidelines for optimizing patient outcomes. The EBP process, first and foremost, promotes the asking of the question, and then utilizes the scientific framework of peer-reviewed literature searches, critical appraisal, and the foundation of nursing knowledge to reach an endpoint that can be reproduced, translated, and shaped into new knowledge.

Because of Florence Nightingale's initial influence, nursing also relies on epidemiologic models of practice and the environment or its variations. When such models are used, cases are tracked, patients/families/communities are treated, and prevention strategies are employed. More recently, nurses within public health are conscious of and employ strategies that consider the entire ecological system to optimize health and prevent or treat illness.

Regardless of the theoretical knowledge base upon which nursing practice is derived, the knowledge fits within the multidimensional nursing process. The nursing process appears linear on first inspection, but is also iterative and incremental, depending upon individual, family, group, community, or population responses.

Evidence-based competencies are foundational to the nursing process. For example, questions regarding clinical practices for the purpose of improving the quality of care may query assessment, diagnosis, planning, outcomes identification, implementation, evaluation, or a combination of these. Describing clinical problems using internal evidence relates to assessment data, diagnosis, and outcomes identification. Evidence-based competencies work hand in hand with outcome measurement, including cost measures (e.g., costs averted, cost savings), nursing-sensitive quality indicators, and the 2001 IOM outcome categories of clinical effectiveness, safety, efficiency, patient-centeredness, timeliness, and equitability (IOM, 2001). Outcome measures may also refer to diagnostic-specific nursing outcomes as stipulated in *Nursing Outcomes Classification* (Moorhead, Johnson, Maas, & Swanson, 2012).

Knowledge translation is also known as evidence-based decision-making, research utilization, innovation diffusion, knowledge transfer, research dissemination, research implementation, and research uptake (Estabrooks et al., 2006, p. 28). Translation of knowledge to practice settings aims to achieve identified outcomes for systems, providers, educators, healthcare consumers, and other stakeholders. This effort continues to be one of the most daunting challenges to registered nurses, but provides exciting opportunities.

Translation of research into practice is a science unto itself, known as translational research. Nurses are at the forefront of this work as they implement evidence-based practices into clinical care, lead research teams to investigate barriers and facilitators of knowledge translation, and advocate at all policy levels for the adoption of these practices throughout the healthcare system. The surge in the scholarly evaluation of evidence-based practice by the expanding ranks of nurses prepared at the doctoral level has contributed to enhanced utilization of evidence-based practice or translation of research into practice.

The failure to employ a theoretically driven knowledge translation plan prevents the development of testable and useful interventions reflecting thoughtful consideration of the nursing process to the target of the intervention. Estabrooks et al. (2006) provide an overview of selected knowledge translation theories spanning the individual healthcare consumer, team, organization, community, and populations. Newhouse (2010) reminds nurses that inclusion of a cost analysis is key when recommending any knowledge translation plan to healthcare consumers or decision-making bodies.

The Where of Nursing Practice

Nursing occurs in any environment where there is a healthcare consumer in need of care, information, or advocacy. The following content describes a sampling of settings and environments for today's evolving and expanding nursing presence. Originally nurses provided nursing services to patients and their families in home settings. Public health nursing resources focused on prevention initiatives and support of community and population health. Establishment of hospitals as inpatient centers for acute care services provided new opportunities for registered nurses. Today home health, post-acute care, assisted living, and long-term care facilities, and community-based living, outpatient, and ambulatory settings are gaining in popularity. This evolution has greater importance as transitions in care, cost reduction measures, financial penalties for adverse outcomes, and healthcare reform initiatives materialize. New technologies have enabled establishment of ambulatory surgical centers and interventional services providers, such as facilities for cardiology and radiology studies and therapies, and infusion and dialysis centers.

Nursing practice in correctional facilities, military organizations, air and ground transport services, and emergency preparedness and disaster support is less commonly identified. Nursing practice in educational settings is represented as school and college health nursing services or academic and professional development and continuing education faculty roles. Other nursing practice settings include occupational health departments, public and private organizations or businesses, faith communities, research and quality improvement organizations, administrative and informatics positions, and entrepreneurial ventures. Smartphone and telehealth technologies, wearable devices and remote monitoring, as well as social media and the Internet, are transforming health care and nursing practice to virtual, "always on" access. Such technology solutions enable nursing practice to move from local settings to national, international, global, and even outer space venues.

Advocacy is fundamental to nursing practice in all settings. Advocacy is "the act or process of pleading for, supporting, recommending a cause or course of action" (ANA, 2015, p. 41). Advocacy occurs at the individual, interpersonal, organization and community, and policy levels (Earp, French, & Gilkey, 2008). At the **individual level**, the nurse engages in informing healthcare consumers so they can consider actions, interventions, or choices in light of their own personal beliefs, attitudes, and knowledge to achieve the desired outcome. Thus the healthcare consumer learns self-management and patient-centered decision-making.

At the **interpersonal level**, the nurse empowers healthcare consumers by providing emotional support, attainment of resources, and necessary help through interactions with families and significant others in their social support network. At the **organization and community level**, the nurse supports cultural transformation of organizations, communities, or populations when present. Registered nurses firmly believe it is their obligation to help improve environmental and societal conditions related to health, wellness, and care of the healthcare consumer. Such issues have included but are not limited to protective labor laws, minimum wage, communicable disease programs, immunizations, well-baby and child care, women's health, violence, reproductive health, and end-of-life care.

Finally, at the **policy level**, the nurse translates the consumer voice into policy and legislation that address such issues as control of healthcare access, regulation of health care, protection of the healthcare consumer, and environmental justice. Thus advocacy also occurs when registered nurses represent professional nursing practice in advocating for the removal of barriers to permit practice to the full extent of their education and training. Registered nurses also advocate as seated members in state and national legislative bodies, IOM committees, and organizational leadership level boards; as they lobby for healthcare issues and resources; and when they join with vulnerable communities fighting industry and dilapidated housing that threatens the health of individuals, group, communities, and populations. Registered nurses are also advocates when addressing malpractice concerns and in their roles as legal nurse consultants or when engaged in legal practice as nurse attorneys.

The nurse understands that "place matters" because of the environmental impact of where people grow, learn, work, and reside. Advocacy, as defined by nursing, can take place wherever healthcare consumers exist or their needs require representation (e.g., streets to the halls of legislatures). There is ample need for professional nurses to continue advocacy and lobbying efforts for the evaluation and restructuring of health care, reimbursement and value of nursing care, funding for nursing education, identifying the role of nurses and nursing in health and medical homes, comparative effectiveness, and advances in health information technology. Nurses will continue to remain strong advocates for healthcare consumers, their care, health care, and the nursing profession.

Healthy Work Environments for Nursing Practice

A healthy work environment is one that is safe, empowering, and satisfying, not merely the absence of real and perceived physical or emotional threats to health, but a place of physical, mental, and social well-being, supporting optimal health and safety. A culture of safety is paramount, in which all leaders, managers, healthcare workers, and ancillary staff have a responsibility as part of the interprofessional team to perform with a sense of professionalism, accountability, transparency, involvement, efficiency, and effectiveness. All must be mindful of the health and safety of both the healthcare consumer and the healthcare worker in any setting providing health care, providing a sense of safety, respect, and empowerment to and for all persons.

Nurses and other healthcare professionals are challenged with the complexities and intensity of work inherent in all healthcare settings. Many factors influence healthcare work environments, including economic challenges, the rapidity with which new information and healthcare technologies are introduced into healthcare settings, demographic shifts, aging and obesity of both the nursing workforce and the general population, the growth of transitional care across all settings, and the impact of healthcare reform. These factors have created significant changes, sometimes perceived as barriers to achieving healthy work environments that support and promote the best patient care and the health and well-being of the nurse.

Safe Patient Handling and Mobility (SPHM)

The establishment of a healthy work environment is predicated on a culture of safety. Nurses in all specialty areas are at varying risk for musculoskeletal and other injuries, especially due to lifting and patient positioning without the right equipment, education, and training. The ANA supports the position that manual patient handling must be eliminated to ensure nurses and other healthcare workers are providing care in a safe work environment (ANA, 2008). The *Safe Patient Handling and Mobility Interprofessional National Standards* (ANA, 2012c) has established standards that address the responsibility of employers and healthcare professionals in establishing an effective safe patient handling and mobility program.

Fatigue in Nursing Practice

The 2015 *Code of Ethics for Nurses with Interpretive Statements* affirms that all nurses, regardless of specialty, have an ethical responsibility to report to work alert, well-rested, and prepared to give safe, quality patient care. Nursing work can be both physically and emotionally exhausting. Long and variable hours, heavy patient loads, and complex care needs that require multi-tasking are just some of the challenges that nurses face every day. Research has demonstrated that fatigue has a major impact on the health and safety of nurses, and on clinical care outcomes. ANA's fatigue position statement (2014c) identifies important strategies that must be implemented by both employers and nurses to reduce the occurrence of fatigue in the workplace.

Workplace Violence and Incivility

Healthcare workers have a fivefold risk of experiencing workplace violence when compared to the overall workforce (National Institute for Occupational Safety and Health, 2013a). The presence of overt and covert workplace violence, bullying, and incivility has a significant impact on both the individual nurse and the overall work environment that includes increased time away from work, higher turnover rates among nurses and other team members, and sub-optimal patient outcomes.

Nurses must advocate for policies and procedures that address the issue of workplace violence and incivility. The American Nurses Association maintains the position that nurses have the right to work in an environment free of abusive behavior and violence (ANA, 2012b). The National Institute for Occupational Safety and Health (NIOSH) provides extensive resources, training, and education specific to nurses to assist in the development of a comprehensive workplace violence prevention program (NIOSH, 2013a).

Optimal Staffing

The issue of optimal staffing has a significant impact on the work environment and continues to be a priority concern of nurses at all levels of practice (ANA, 2014a). Economic constraints, shortages of qualified staff, shortened lengths of stay, and patient care needs that are increasingly complex, are all factors that contribute to the challenges inherent in creating and sustaining staffing models that promote optimal staffing for safe patient care. ANA's *Principles for Nurse Staffing* (ANA, 2012a) provides a framework to assist nurses at all levels in evaluating and revising current staffing models to improve the work environment for nurses, and ultimately, to improve outcomes of clinical care. This framework includes principles related to:

- Healthcare consumers
- Registered nurses and other staff
- Organization and workplace culture
- The practice environment
- Staffing evaluation

Optimal staffing is a critical component of a healthy work environment. Contemporary staffing models should include elements that support team-based care, which has been identified as a highly effective model that promotes safe, effective, and efficient care (Agency for Healthcare Research and Quality, 2008). Innovative strategies that incorporate the best evidence and a collaborative team approach provide the greatest opportunity to overcome barriers and improve nurse satisfaction and patient care. Nurses who work as independent contractors in homes and other uncontrolled settings are responsible for avoiding fatigue and accessing team members and other resources as needed.

Supports for Healthy Work Environments

The following initiatives, frameworks, models, and constructs demonstrate characteristics important to the development and maintenance of an exemplary work environment.

American Nurses Association (ANA)

The initial ANA Healthy Nurse™ framework began in 2009. The definition and constructs are as follows: ANA defines the healthy nurse as

one who actively focuses on creating and maintaining a balance and synergy of physical, intellectual, emotional, social, spiritual, personal and professional well-being. Healthy nurses live life to the fullest capacity, across the wellness–illness continuum, as they become stronger role models, advocates, and educators, personally, for their families, their communities and work environments, and ultimately for their patients. (ANA, 2013b)

The five Healthy Nurse™ constructs include:

Calling to Care: Caring is the interpersonal, compassionate offering of self by which the healthy nurse builds relationships with patients and their families, while helping them meet their physical, emotional, and spiritual goals, for all ages, in all healthcare settings, across the care continuum.

Priority to Self-Care: Self-care and supportive environments enable the healthy nurse to increase the ability to effectively manage the physical and emotional stressors of the work and home environments.

Opportunity to Role Model: The healthy nurse confidently recognizes and identifies personal health challenges in themselves and their patients, thereby enabling them and their patients to overcome the challenge in a collaborative, non-accusatory manner.

Responsibility to Educate: Using non-judgmental approaches, considering adult learning patterns and readiness to change, the healthy nurse empowers themselves and others by sharing health, safety, wellness knowledge, skills, resources, and attitudes.

Authority to Advocate: The healthy nurse is empowered to advocate on numerous levels, including personally, interpersonally, within the work environment and the community, and at the local, state, and national levels in policy development and advocacy.

American Nurses Credentialing Center (ANCC Programs)
THE MAGNET RECOGNITION PROGRAM

The Magnet Recognition Program® provides a framework for practice that has a significant impact on the professional nursing work environment. To achieve and maintain Magnet recognition, Magnet®-designated facilities must demonstrate the following model components:

Transformational Leadership: Transformational leaders have the ability to articulate a strong vision that aligns strategic goals across the organization. They inspire their followers to succeed by empowering them to achieve professional goals and developing them professionally into leaders.

Structural Empowerment: Structural empowerment is achieved by developing structures and processes that support a decentralized environment, include a shared governance and decision-making framework, support lifelong learning, professional development, certification and academic advancement, and promotes the voice of nursing by ensuring that nurses, including the Chief Nursing Officer (CNO), are included in decision-making at all levels of the organization.

Exemplary Professional Practice: This demonstrates what professional nursing practice can achieve with structures and processes that support professional roles of the nurse as consultant, teacher, and interprofessional team member. Exemplary professional practice also promotes professional models of care, autonomy, quality improvement, and quality of care.

New Knowledge, Innovation, and Improvements: To evolve and innovate, organizations must proactively integrate research and best evidence into clinical and operational practice.

Empirical Outcomes: Recognizing that outcomes are essential to establishing and maintaining organizational excellence, the 2008 Magnet Manual reflected that significant shift in focus and included outcome standards that have carried through to the 2014 Magnet Manual. Nearly half of the standards in the current manual are outcome-focused. (ANCC, 2014)

PATHWAY TO EXCELLENCE PROGRAM

The American Nurses Credentialing Center developed the Pathway to Excellence® Program to recognize healthcare organizations that demonstrate successful implementation of the Pathway to Excellence® structure and process standards that promote a healthy work environment and meet the Pathway Practice Standards:

1. Nurses control the practice of nursing

2. The work environment is safe and healthy

3. Systems are in place to address patient care and practice concerns

4. Orientation prepares nurses for the work environment

5. The CNO is qualified and participates in all levels of the organization

6. Professional development is provided and used

7. Equitable compensation is provided

8. Nurses are recognized for achievements

9. A balanced lifestyle is encouraged

10. Collaborative relationships are valued and supported

11. Nurse managers are competent and accountable

12. A quality program and evidence-based practice are used. (ANCC, 2012)

American Association of Critical-Care Nurses Standards

The American Association of Critical-Care Nurses has identified six standards for establishing and maintaining healthy work environments that remain unchanged today:

Skilled Communication: Nurses must be as proficient in communication skills as they are in clinical skills.

True Collaboration: Nurses must be relentless in pursuing and fostering a sense of team and partnership across all disciplines.

Effective Decision-making: Nurses are seen as valued and committed partners in making policy, directing and evaluating clinical care, and leading organizational operations.

Appropriate Staffing: Staffing must ensure the effective match between healthcare consumer needs and nurse competencies.

Meaningful Recognition: Nurses must be recognized and must recognize others for the value each brings to the work of the organization.

Authentic Leadership: Nurse leaders must fully embrace the imperative of a healthy work environment, authentically live it, and engage others in achieving it. (American Association of Colleges of Nursing, 2005, p. 13)

American Holistic Nurses Association (AHNA Core Values)

The AHNA/ANA's *Holistic Nursing: Scope and Standards of Practice, Second Edition* (2013) includes five core values that promote the importance of caring for oneself, and the creation of a therapeutic environment:

Core Value 1. Holistic Philosophy, Theories, and Ethics

Core Value 2. Holistic Caring Process

Core Value 3. Holistic Communication, Therapeutic Healing Environment, and Cultural Diversity

Core Value 4. Holistic Education and Research

Core Value 5. Holistic Nurse Self-Reflection and Self-Care

Samueli Institute

The Samueli Institute (2010) has conducted extensive research on healing environments and has identified four domains that comprise an optimal work environment:

Domain 1. Internal Environments: Focus on the health and wellness of self, intentionality in caring, and personal wholeness.

Domain 2. Interpersonal Environments: Focus on the cultivation of healing relationships, both collegial and at the organizational level.

Domain 3. Behavioral Environments: Focus on healthy lifestyle and team-based, person- and family-centered care.

Domain 4. External Environments: Focus on actions that support external healing environments and a healthy planet.

High-Performing Interprofessional Teams

Nurses are familiar with collaborative work groups that foster collegial relationships focused on sharing of specialized skills and information. In this paradigm, clinicians are rewarded for individual performance rather than team-based results. This does not yet reflect an evolution to high-performing interprofessional teams: interprofessional competency in health care has been defined as:

integrated enactment of knowledge, skills, and values/attitudes that define working together across the professions, with other health care workers, and with patients, along with families and communities, as appropriate to improve health outcomes in specific care contexts. (Interprofessional Education Collaborative Expert Panel, 2011, p. 2)

The Expert Panel identified four interprofessional collaborative practice domains, which are both community and population-oriented and patient- and family-centered. These competency domains include:

- Values/Ethics for Interprofessional Practice
- Interprofessional Teamwork and Team-based Practice
- Interprofessional Communication Practices Roles, and
- Responsibilities for Collaborative Practice

The Institute of Medicine (IOM) identifies multiple issues inherent in any care delivery model that does not include high performance teamwork, including adverse events related to inadequate communication and handoffs, and the potential for duplication and waste resulting in higher healthcare costs (Mitchell et al., 2012). A study performed at the Massachusetts Institute of Technology identified effective communication patterns as the single most critical factor in determining the degree of success of work teams (Pentland, 2012).

The Agency for Healthcare Research and Quality (AHRQ) has identified Team-based Care as a highly effective care delivery model that promotes safe, effective, and efficient health care (AHRQ, 2008). Care coordination has been identified as a "traditional strength of the nursing profession" (IOM, 2010), and nurses have been identified as having the "critical history, knowledge, and expertise needed to assure that care coordination achieves the goals set forth for it in the national quality agenda" (Lamb, 2014, p. 3). Nurses have demonstrated the positive impact of nurse-led teams (Watts et al., 2009).

Many reference Tuckman's 1965 *Forming, Storming, Norming, Performing Model* when describing the characteristics and evolution of a successful high performing team (Eyre, n.d.). He identified that high performing teams complete four developmental stages: forming, storming, norming, and performing, and added a fifth stage, adjourning, in the 1970s. RNs and APRNs are often key contributors and leaders in each stage.

Key Influences on the Quality and Environment of Nursing Practice

Many organizations seek to influence society and nursing through similar and/or shared purposes, goals, and agendas. Each nurse must be aware of historical, contemporary, and future internal or external influences that can impact nursing practice and those served. Validation through scientific, nursing-focused inquiry enables nursing practice to proactively evolve to address global influences. Such influences include, but are not limited to, the Tri-Regulator Collaborative, Institute of Medicine, the National Council of State Boards of Nursing, the Robert Wood Johnson Foundation (RWJF), and others.

The recently established Tri-Regulator Collaborative is comprised of

> the leading organizations representing the licensing boards of the United States that regulate the practice of medicine, pharmacy, and nursing, the Federation of State Medical Boards, National Association of Boards of Pharmacy, and National Council of State Boards of Nursing. (Tri-Regulator Collaborative, 2014)

Its aim is to improve the quality of health care in the United States through a team-based approach to patient care and it is projected to have increasing impact on professional practice and education.

In an article released by the Robert Wood Johnson Foundation, October 2014, Melanie Dreher, PhD, RN, FAAN, is quoted as saying:

> Nursing is the largest and most trusted healthcare profession, and nurses spend more time with patients than other providers and see patients in their broader environments—in their communities and homes and with family members.... More nurse leaders are needed in all sectors to share their unique insights into factors that affect health and health care and the best ways to engage caregivers and loved ones in patient care. No one understands patients—the person part of the patient—the way nurses do. (Dreher, 2014)

To address issues in health care, the Institute of Medicine, a branch of the National Academy of Sciences, commissions reports on scientific topics. Its reports and other publications are most often directed toward universal healthcare practice and sometimes explicitly to nursing, and provide a framework for positive change in healthcare services.

In 1999, the Quality of Health Care in America Committee released the first and arguably most pivotal report, *To Err Is Human: Building a Safer Health System*, which suggested that harm done to healthcare consumers in a profession that strives to "First, do no harm" is unacceptable. One of the most influential and paradigm-shifting conclusions of the report was that individuals and reckless behavior played only a small part in patient safety violations, and that faulty systems in which people were set up for failure were more problematic.

A second report by the committee in 2001, *Crossing the Quality Chasm: A New Health System for the 21st Century*, urged a fundamental, sweeping redesign of the entire health system. Incremental change was not enough. The committee suggested that such a system would not only improve patient safety and quality outcomes, but would also retain more health professionals who felt their contributions were making a satisfactory impact on those to whom they provide care.

Keeping Patients Safe: Transforming the Work Environment of Nurses is a key report that considers how nurses' interactions with their workplace help or hinder patient care. The report reviews evidence on the work and work environments of nurses and takes into account the behavioral traits of nurses, the organizational practices and culture, and the structural and engineering traits of the workplace. The report identified leadership and management, the workforce, work processes, and organizational culture as the components of the workplace most influential on nursing and patient outcomes. This report proposes changes to those components that would lead to better outcomes for patients and nurses (IOM, 2004). To date, few work environments have achieved all the IOM recommendations from 2004. The healthcare industry must alter the work environment of nurses to allow them to meet their social responsibility for healthcare consumer safety.

The Future of Nursing: Leading Change, Advancing Health (IOM, 2010) and the subsequent Future of Nursing Campaign are providing strategies for nursing and nurses to become more influential, visibly active, outcome-oriented, and positioned in strategic positions in the public arena. The first recommendation in the report addresses the need to remove scope of practice barriers. Nurses are called to engage in activities that target major stakeholders, such as Congress, Centers for Medicare and Medicaid Services, and state legislative and regulatory bodies, to remove barriers and enable nurses to practice at the highest level of their education and training and promote enhanced consumer access to quality health care.

Action related to nursing education has created momentum and new partnerships between undergraduate programs and academia and practice partnerships. Revised goals in nursing education include eventual achievement of a doctorate in nursing practice or a Doctor of Philosophy in Nursing as the terminal degree for the profession. This report specifically recommends increasing the amount of nurses with Bachelor of Science in Nursing (BSN) degrees to 80% by 2020 (Recommendation 4) and to double the amount of doctorally prepared nurses by 2020 (Recommendation 5). A renewed respect for lifelong learning has been developed in the various communications provided to the profession of nursing.

Additionally, *The Future of Nursing* has identified, through survey and questioning, the lack of registered nurses who serve on opinion-generating and policy-making boards. Such boards are responsible for provision of direction for the nation's health care and rely on the Affordable Care Act and Medicaid Expansion as a formidable plank for their decision-making process.

IOM reports that continue to influence nursing practice include others, such as *Dying in America: Improving Quality and Honoring Individual Preferences Near the End of Life*; *Best Care at Lower Cost: The Path to Continuously Learning Health Care in America*; *Primary Care and Public Health: Exploring Integration to Improve Population Health*; and *Health IT and Patient Safety: Building Safer Systems for Better Care*. Nurses are increasingly important participants and contributors in the work of the IOM.

Healthy People 2020 highlights the importance of addressing the social determinants of health identified as these five key areas: economic stability, education, social and community context, health and health care, and neighborhood and built environments. Each determinant is characterized by a number of critical components and key issues. More details are available at http://www.healthypeople.gov/2020/topics-objectives/topic/social-determinants-health.

Although nursing defines its own scope and standards of practice in care delivery systems and education environments, the profession is greatly enhanced through the contributions of these external influences. The external influences affecting nursing are too numerous to list but each can serve as a catalyst for collaboration, promote partnerships in healthcare delivery, and reflect substantive support for nurses and nursing practice.

Societal, Cultural, and Ethical Dimensions Describe the Why and How of Nursing

The need for health care is universal and transcends differences with respect to the culture, values, and preferences of the individual, family, group, community, and population. Diversity characterizes today's healthcare environment. Nursing is responsive to the changing needs of society and the expanding knowledge base of its theoretical and scientific domains. One of nursing's objectives is to achieve positive healthcare consumer outcomes that maximize one's quality of life across the entire life span. To effectively promote meaningful outcomes, nurses must embrace that diversity and engage in culturally congruent practice.

Culturally congruent practice is the application of evidence-based nursing that is in agreement with the preferred cultural values, beliefs, worldview, and practices of the healthcare consumer and other stakeholders. Cultural competence represents the process by which nurses demonstrate culturally congruent practice. Nurses design and direct culturally congruent practice and services for diverse consumers to improve access, promote positive outcomes, and reduce disparities.

A number of theories and models outline how culturally congruent practice may be implemented. Examples include, but are not limited to:

- Andrews/Boyle Transcultural Interprofessional Practice Model (TIP), developed by Margaret M. Andrews and Joyceen S. Boyle (Andrews & Boyle, 2015 in press)

- The Process of Cultural Competence in the Delivery of Health Services, Model, developed by Josepha Campinha-Bacote (Campinha-Bacote, 2011b)

- Culture Care Diversity and Universality, developed by Madeleine Leininger. [Leininger & McFarland (2002), and McFarland & Wehbe-Alamah (2015)]

- Giger & Davidhizar's Transcultural Assessment Model, developed by Joyce Newman Giger & Ruth Elaine Davidhizar (Giger & Davidhizar, 2008)

- Jeffreys's Cultural Competence and Confidence (CCC) Model, developed by Marianne R. Jeffreys (Jeffreys, 2010)

- Purnell Model for Cultural Competence, developed by Larry Purnell (Purnell, 2013)

- The HEALTH Traditions Model, developed by Rachel E. Spector, includes three assessment tools and one interview guide (Spector, 2013).

Some of these authors have provided tools and guides for implementation of culturally congruent practice. For example, many nurses have found the mnemonic ASKED (**A**wareness, **S**kill, **K**nowledge, **E**ncounters, **D**esire) a helpful resource (http://www.transculturalcare.net/cultural_competence_model.htm). Campinha-Bacote used a case study (Vignette: "To Coin, or Not to Coin: That Is the Question") to demonstrate how nurses can partner with consumers in resolving cultural conflict between the consumer's culture and the provider's evidence-based practice guidelines (2011b). See Appendix F for further resources about culturally congruent practice.

Registered nurses enable and promote the interprofessional and comprehensive care provided by healthcare professionals, paraprofessionals, and volunteers. Nurses also engage in consultation and collaboration with other healthcare colleagues to inform decision-making and planning to meet healthcare consumer needs. Registered nurses often participate in interprofessional teams in which the overlapping skills complement each team member's individual efforts.

Registered nurses, regardless of specialty, role, or setting, are accountable for nursing judgments made and actions taken in the course of their nursing practice. Therefore, the registered nurse is responsible for assessing one's own individual competence and is committed to the process of lifelong learning. Registered nurses develop and maintain current knowledge and skills through formal and continuing education and must be encouraged to always seek and maintain certification when it is available in their areas of practice.

Registered nurses and members of various professions exchange knowledge and ideas about how to deliver safe and high-quality health care, resulting in overlaps and constantly changing professional practice boundaries. In accordance with recommendations from professional organizations that team-based care improves safety, satisfaction, quality, and efficiency, nurses are contributing to and leading initiatives in the provision of team-based patient-centered care and development of a collegial work environment (IECEP, 2011). Such interprofessional team collaboration involves recognition of the expertise of others within and outside one's profession and referral to those providers when appropriate. Such collaboration also involves some shared functions and a common focus on one overall mission. By necessity, nursing's scope of practice has flexible boundaries.

Registered nurses regularly evaluate safety, effectiveness, and cost in the planning and delivery of nursing care. Given the current economic environment, nurses strive to be fiscally responsible in the allocation and utilization of resources. Nurses recognize resources are limited and unequally distributed, and the potential for better access to care requires innovative approaches, such as treating healthcare consumers in nurse-managed healthcare centers and telehealth services. As members of a profession, registered nurses promote equitable distribution, access to, and availability of healthcare services throughout the nation and the world.

Legislative changes have expanded the role of nurses as advocates in giving voice to ethical issues for the profession and those for whom they provide care. Issues originating at the bedside become evident as patients progress through the continuum of care. Nurses engage in discussion of these issues in diverse consumer and professional media. As new challenges arise in response to advances in technology, changing roles, and regulatory amendments, nurses promote discussion of patient-centered care, achieve consensus for decision-making, empower the community to action, and mentor development of self-care skills based on the profession's responsibility to the health and well-being of humanity.

Registered nurses are bound by a professional code of ethics (ANA, 2015) and regulate themselves as individuals through a collegial review of practice. Such a review fosters the refinement of knowledge, skills, and clinical decision-making at all levels and in all areas of nursing practice. Self-regulation by the profession of nursing assures quality of performance, which is the heart of nursing's social contract (ANA, 2010b).

Model of Professional Nursing Practice Regulation

In 2006, the Model of Professional Nursing Practice Regulation (see Figure 2) emerged from ANA work and informed the discussions of specialty nursing and advanced practice registered nurse practice. The lowest level in the model represents the responsibility of the professional nurse and the professional and specialty nursing organizations to their members and the public to define the scope and standards of nursing practice.

FIGURE 2. Model of Professional Nursing Practice Regulation

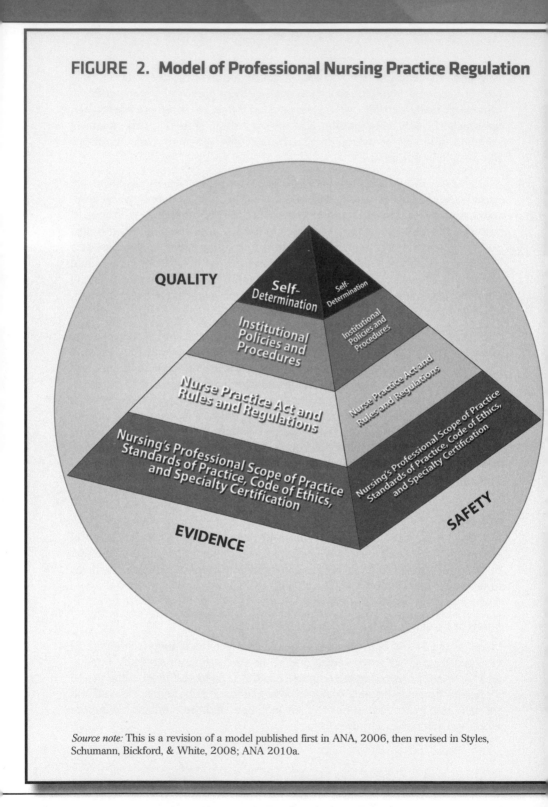

Source note: This is a revision of a model published first in ANA, 2006, then revised in Styles, Schumann, Bickford, & White, 2008; ANA 2010a.

*Serif text denotes the "what" of each tier. **Sans serif** text denotes the "who" of each tier. For more about the "what" of nursing, see pg. 7. For more about the "who" of nursing, see pg. 38.*

Peak: Self-Determination

This peak represents self-regulation and self-determination by each individual nurse in exercising judgments based upon the integration of content, decisions, and actions from the three lower tiers. The resultant demonstrated behaviors reflect responsible and accountable nursing practice decisions culminating in safe, quality, evidence-based practice. The peak culminates in a point directed upward synonymous to an illuminating path from Nightingale's lamp to emphasize continued potential toward a higher level of individual professional practice regulation.

Participants: Registered nurses, graduate-level prepared registered nurses, and advanced practice registered nurses*.

Institutional Policies and Procedures

Regulation at the institutional, organizational, or systems level occurs through the established policies, procedures, and governing statements that influence and direct nursing practice and its environment.

Participants: Institutions, organizations, entities, and systems where nurses are present, chief nursing officers and executives, healthcare administrators, nursing managers, nursing supervisors, registered nurses, graduate-level prepared registered nurses, advanced practice registered nurses*, third-party reimbursement entities, and academic institutions.

Nurse Practice Act and Rules and Regulations

Legislative and regulatory authorities govern through nurse practice acts, statute, code, and regulation administered by state boards of nursing and exemplified by licensure status.

Participants: State or territorial boards of nursing, legislators, lobbyists, National Council of State Boards of Nursing, healthcare advocacy groups, healthcare consumers as voters, political action committees, registered nurses, graduate-leve prepared registered nurses, and advanced practice registered nurses.

Foundation: Nursing's Professional Scope of Practice, Standards of Practice, Code of Ethics, and Specialty Certification

ANA's *Nursing: Scope and Standards of Practice* and *Code of Ethics for Nurses with Interpretive Statements* are essential professional resources that collectively guide nursing practice in all roles and settings. Compliance with the *Code of Ethics for Nurses with Interpretive Statements* and identified standards of practice and accompanying competencies reflects the expected level of competence of all nurses. Specialty certification provides additional verification and validation of competence for a focused body of knowledge and associated skill sets of practice.

Participants: American Nurses Association, credentialing and educational organizations, professional nursing organizations, healthcare consumers as care partners, registered nurses, graduate-level prepared registered nurses, and advanced practice registered nurses*.

(*The APRN direct care roles include certified registered nurse anesthetists, certified nurse midwives, clinical nurse specialists, and certified nurse practitioners.)

The next level up in the pyramid represents the regulation provided by the nurse practice acts, rules, and regulations in the pertinent licensing jurisdictions. Institutional policies and procedures provide further considerations in the next level of regulation of nursing practice for the registered nurse and advanced practice registered nurse.

Note the highest level is that of self-determination by the nurse upon consideration of all the other levels of input about professional nursing practice regulation. Each level builds on the lower ones, ascending in order of impact from the foundation to the peak. The concepts of Safety, Quality, and Evidence are integral to all four levels, and are represented as three sides of a tetrahedron. The goals of individualized professional self-determination are positive patient outcomes and healthcare outcomes resulting from safe, quality, and evidenced-based nursing practice decisions.

The Code of Ethics for Nurses

The *Code of Ethics for Nurses with Interpretive Statements* ("The Code"; ANA, 2015) serves as the ethical framework in nursing regardless of practice setting or role, and provides guidance for the future. The nine provisions explicate key ethical concepts and actions for all nurses in all settings.

> The *Code of Ethics for Nurses with Interpretive Statements* arises from the long, distinguished, and enduring moral tradition of modern nursing in the United States. It is foundational to nursing theory, practice, and praxis in its expression of the values, virtues, and obligations that shape, guide, and inform nursing as a profession. It establishes the ethical standard for the profession and provides a guide for nurses to use in ethical analysis and decision-making. (ANA, 2015, p. vii)

The Code also describes the ethical characteristics of the professional nurse:

> Individuals who become nurses, as well as the professional organizations that represent them, are expected not only to adhere to the values, moral norms, and ideals of the profession but also to embrace them as a part of what it means to be a nurse. The ethical tradition of nursing is self-reflective, enduring, and distinctive. A code of ethics for the nursing profession makes explicit the primary obligations, values, and ideals of the profession. It provides normative, applied moral guidance for nurses in terms of what they ought to do, be, and seek. The values and obligations in the *Code of Ethics for Nurses* apply to nurses in all roles, in all forms of practice, and in all settings. In fact, it informs every aspect of the nurse's life. (ANA, 2015, p. vii)

Detailed descriptive interpretive statements for each of the nine provisions (below) of the Code are available at http://www.nursingworld.org/codeofethics:

Provision 1. The nurse practices with compassion and respect for the inherent dignity, worth, and unique attributes of every person.

Provision 2. The nurse's primary commitment is to the patient, whether an individual, family, group, community, or population.

Provision 3. The nurse promotes, advocates for, and protects the rights, health, and safety of the patient.

Provision 4. The nurse has authority, accountability, and responsibility for nursing practice; makes decisions; and takes action consistent with the obligation to promote health and to provide optimal care.

Provision 5. The nurse owes the same duties to self as to others, including the responsibility to promote health and safety, preserve wholeness of character and integrity, maintain competence, and continue personal and professional growth.

Provision 6. The nurse, through individual and collective effort, establishes, maintains, and improves the ethical environment of the work setting and conditions of employment that are conducive to safe, quality health care.

Provision 7. The nurse, in all roles and settings, advances the profession through research and scholarly inquiry, professional standards development, and the generation of both nursing and health policy.

Provision 8. The nurse collaborates with other health professionals and the public to protect human rights, promote health diplomacy, and reduce health disparities.

Provision 9. The profession of nursing, collectively through its professional organizations, must articulate nursing values, maintain the integrity of the profession, and integrate principles of social justice into nursing and health policy.

Specialty Practice in Nursing

The continuation of the profession depends on the education of nurses, appropriate organization of nursing services, continued expansion of nursing knowledge, and the development and adoption of policies. Nursing first expanded into public health interventions on behalf of at-risk communities and vulnerable populations. In 1893, Lillian Wald pioneered public health nursing at the Henry Street Settlement House in New York City. In 1899, Teacher's College at Columbia University offered the first university program for graduate nurses to specialize in public health nursing (Stewart, 1948). An editorial in the *American Journal of Nursing* in 1911 pointed out the urgent demand for nurses who could teach others and organize a whole community.

In the mid-20th century and beyond, advances in medical treatment and healthcare technology led to the evolution of other nursing specialties. Such initiatives demand that registered nurses be adequately prepared for these nursing specialties. Specialized education, training, and certification ensued in both traditional and newer areas of clinical practice as nurses evolved from novice to expert clinicians.

Specialty nurses collaborate, consult, and serve as liaisons, bridging the role of the professional registered nurse and those of other professionals, and subsequently help to delineate nursing's role in society. The 2008 APRN Consensus Model provided clarity about the preparation and identification of advanced practice registered nurses who acquire specialized knowledge and skills through graduate-level education in their selected specialty areas. APRNs must achieve specific certifications and are recognized by their respective licensing jurisdictions for the advanced practice registered nurse titles of CNS, CNP, CRNA, CNM.

Some specialties reflect the intersection of nursing's body of knowledge and that of another profession or discipline, directly influence nursing practice, and support direct care delivery to healthcare consumers by registered nurses. Many nurses have completed graduate-level educational preparation for practice in informatics, public health, education, administration, and other specialties that are essential to advancing the public's health and focus on supporting, informing, and guiding care activities and decision-making. In most states these specialty practices do not require regulatory recognition beyond the registered nurse license granted by state boards of nursing.

Competencies in individual specialty areas of practice may be defined by separate specialty scope and standards documents authored by specialty nursing associations. Many specialty nursing organizations recognize individual expertise through national certification in the specialty.

Professional Registered Nurses Today: The Who of Nursing
Statistical Snapshot

Registered nurses, including advanced practice registered nurses, comprise the largest sector of licensed providers in the U.S. healthcare workforce. Nursing practice, while difficult to comprehensively delimit, consists of both clinical and indirect care that include, but are not limited to: direct patient care, public health and population-based care, school nursing, administration, education, informatics, research, consultation, entrepreneurship, and public policy development. Some nurses function in one of these practice areas, while others practice in two or more.

Although nurses must be licensed and thus regulated by each state, significant barriers prevent determination of the total supply of registered nurses practicing in the United States. The current estimate of over 3.4 million registered nurses reflects the dated projection from the 2008 National Sample Survey of Registered Nurses (HRSA, 2010) and an updated analysis and extrapolation (McMenamin, 2015). The continued lack of an accurate and reliable methodology with which to measure the dynamic and fluid number of registered nurses serves as the greatest constraint in confirming the numbers and characteristics of today's nursing constituency. Currently, not all states report information about the number of actively licensed registered nurses to the National Council of State Boards of Nursing's information system that is programmed to identify individuals with active licensure in more than one regulatory jurisdiction.

Another barrier exists as the result of complexities in the employment patterns of registered nurses. Registered nurses may work full-time or part-time in one or more clinical care positions, academic institutions, healthcare and non-health institutions, or other venues. For example, the Occupational Employment Statistics (OES) program of the Bureau of Labor Statistics (BLS) conducts a semi-annual mail survey of employers designed to produce estimates of employment and wages for more than 800 specific occupations. The most recent data published from this survey are for May 2013. The OES survey covers all full- and part-time wage and salary workers in nonfarm industries. The survey does not include the self-employed, owners and partners in unincorporated firms, workers in private households, or unpaid family workers. The survey also does not include persons employed by the U.S. military.

Some registered nurses move from performing registered nurse clinical care functions into management, business, teaching, or other positions where their knowledge and skills as registered nurses are required but where those new positions are no longer classified by the BLS as registered nursing. Some registered nurses leave the profession yet maintain an active registered nurse license. As a result, the OES underestimates the total employment of registered nurses per se because some registered nurses will be classified as managers, administrators, professors, etc. The OES estimates the number of registered nurses who work predominantly within the registered nurses occupational description to be 2,687,310 in May 2014 (U.S. Bureau of Labor Statistics, 2014).

Since 2012, BLS has also published estimates with respect to nurse practitioners (NPs), certified registered nurse anesthetists (CRNAs), and certified nurse midwives (CNMs). Note the clinical nurse specialist category is not identified in the 2012 BLS publication. The OES data collected for the three employed APRN roles are the same as those collected for employed RNs. A key issue is whether the employers characterize their APRN employees as APRNs rather than RNs. Many NPs, for example, remain in job listings that combine all RNs and APRNs in a single "nurse" category. Such nurses are included in the RN estimates. The single best example of such mislabeling and under-reporting is the federal government. The Office of Personnel Management reports there are no NPs employed by the federal government, although the Department of Veterans Affairs has indicated that in May 2013, there were 4,734 NPs employed at the Veterans Administration. The Office of Personnel Management (OPM), which supplies the official employment statistics to BLS, does not have a category for NPs.

The U.S. Bureau of Labor Statistics also produces demand projections for employment numbers for hundreds of occupations. Their new projections cover 2012–2022. BLS projects 555,100 RNs and APRNs will retire or otherwise leave the labor force by 2022. This tsunami of retirements reflects several historical factors associated with the Baby Boom, Title VIII funding variations, and changes in career opportunities for women that occurred in the 1970s and 1980s. In addition to the replacement needs, BLS also projects increases in demand for an additional 574,400 RNs and APRNs, yielding total projected openings of 1.13 million.

The demand for nurses has been expressed in various ways, including the availability of open job postings for registered nurses, the geographical distribution of registered nurses, and the percent of nursing school applicants who are rejected for admission due to unavailability of qualified nursing faculty. Furthermore, the future demand for registered nurses has been difficult to estimate as a result of health policy reform, shifting preferences for entry-level nursing education, and several other factors, most of which have yet to be identified.

This inability to accurately determine both the supply and demand of registered nurses results in both over-reporting and under-reporting of registered nurse workforce shortage and surplus. What most registered nurse workforce analysts can agree upon is that shortages and surpluses may be in existence simultaneously within the United States, depending on geography, type of practice, local fluctuations in population healthcare needs, state and institutional barriers to nursing scope of practice, and other factors.

Licensure and Education of Registered Nurses

The registered nurse is licensed and authorized by a state, commonwealth, or territory to practice nursing. Professional licensure of the healthcare professions is established by each jurisdiction to protect the public safety and authorize the practice of that profession. Because of this, the requirements for RN and APRN licensure vary widely.

The registered nurse is educationally prepared for competent practice at the entry level upon graduation from an accredited diploma, associate degree, baccalaureate, or master's degree nursing program and is qualified by national examination (National Council Licensure Examination for Registered Nurses, known as NCLEX-RN) for RN licensure. The licensing jurisdiction then grants the legal title of registered nurse, shortened to RN, allowing nurses to use the RN credential after their name as long as their license remains in an active status. ANA has consistently affirmed the baccalaureate degree in nursing as the preferred educational preparation for entry into nursing practice.

The registered nurse is educated in the art and science of nursing, with the goal of helping individuals, families, groups, communities, and populations attain, maintain, and restore health whenever possible. Experienced nurses may become proficient in one or more practice areas or roles and may elect to concentrate on care of the healthcare consumer in clinical nursing practice specialties. Others influence nursing and support the direct clinical care rendered to healthcare consumers. Credentialing is one form of acknowledging such specialized knowledge and experience. Credentialing organizations may mandate specific nursing educational requirements, as well as timely demonstrations of knowledge and experience in specialty practice.

Registered nurses may pursue advanced academic studies to prepare for specialization in practice. Educational requirements vary by specialty and academic educational program. New models for educational preparation are evolving in response to the changing healthcare, education, and regulatory practice environments. A continued commitment to the nursing profession requires registered nurses to remain involved in continuous learning, thereby strengthening individual practice within varied settings (see Standard 12. Education on page 76). Participation in civic activities, membership in and support of professional associations, collective bargaining, and workplace advocacy also demonstrate professional commitment. Nurses commit to their profession by utilizing their skills, knowledge, and abilities to act as visionaries, promoting safe practice environments, and supporting resourceful, accessible, and cost-effective delivery of health care to serve the ever-changing needs of the population.

Registered nurses who pursue advanced education at the graduate or doctoral level may select programs and courses of study that do not prepare them for licensure and recognition as advanced practice registered nurses. Because these graduate-level prepared registered nurses may be expected to demonstrate additional competencies beyond those of registered nurses, such competencies are clearly identified in the accompanying standards of professional practice section of this resource.

Advanced Practice Registered Nurse Roles

Another evolution of nursing practice was the development of educational programs to prepare nurses for advanced practice in direct care roles. These APRN roles include certified registered nurse anesthetists (CRNAs), certified nurse midwives (CNMs), clinical nurse specialists (CNSs), and certified nurse practitioners (CNPs). Each has a unique history and context, but all share a focus on direct care to individual healthcare consumers. *Advanced Practice Registered Nurse* is a regulatory title and includes the four roles listed above. State law and regulation further define criteria for licensure for the designated advanced practice registered nurse roles. The need to ensure healthcare consumer safety and access to APRNs by aligning education, accreditation, licensure, and certification is shown in the *Consensus Model for APRN Regulation: Licensure, Accreditation, Certification, and Education* (APRN Joint Dialogue Group, 2008).

In addition to the licensure, accreditation, certification, and education (LACE) requirements for advanced practice registered nurses outlined in the Consensus Model, the following professional, accreditation, and certification organizations address standards and competencies for each advanced practice role:

- Accreditation Commission for Midwifery Education: *Criteria for Programmatic Accreditation* (December 2009, revised June 2013).

- American Association of Nurse Anesthetists: *Scope of Nurse Anesthesia Practice* (2013), and *Standards for Nurse Anesthesia Practice* (2013)
  http://www.aana.com/resources2/professionalpractice/Pages/Professional-Practice-Manual.aspx#scope.

- American Association of Nurse Practitioners: *Standards of Practice for Nurse Practitioners* (2013).

- American Nurses Credentialing Center
  http://www.nursecredentialing.org.

- American College of Nurse-Midwives: *Core Competencies for Basic Midwifery Practice* (June 2012)
  http://www.midwife.org/ACNM/files/ccLibraryFiles/Filename/000000002730/Core%20Competencies%20June%202012.pdf.

- *Standards for the Practice of Midwifery* (2009)
  http://www.midwife.org/ACNM/files/ccLibraryFiles/
  Filename/000000000270/Standards_for_Practice_of_
  Midwifery_12_09_001.pdf.

- Council on Accreditation of Nurse Anesthesia Educational Programs:
  Standards for Accreditation of Nurse Anesthesia Educational Programs
  (2014)
  http://home.coa.us.com/accreditation/Pages/Accreditation-Policies-
  Procedures-and-Standards.aspx.

- National Organization of Nurse Practitioner Faculties: *Domains and
  Core Competencies of Nurse Practitioner Practice* (2012). Available at
  http://c.ymcdn.com/sites/www.nonpf.org/resource/resmgr/compe-
  tencies/npcorecompetenciesfinal2012.pdf.

- *Population-focused Nurse Practitioner Competencies. Family/
  Across the Lifespan, Neonatal, Pediatric Acute Care, Pediatric
  Primary Care, Psychiatric-Mental Health, and Women's Health/
  Gender-Specific.* Population Focused Competencies Task Force
  (2013). Available at
  http://c.ymcdn.com/sites/www.nonpf.org/resource/resmgr/
  Competencies/CompilationPopFocusComps2013.pdf.

- National Association of Clinical Nurse Specialists:

  — *Organizing Framework and CNS Core Competencies* (2010)

  — *Core Practice Doctorate Clinical Nurse Specialist (CNS)
    Competencies* (2009), http://www.nacns.org.

Professional Competence in Nursing Practice

The public has a right to expect registered nurses to demonstrate professional competence throughout their careers. The registered nurse is individually responsible and accountable for maintaining professional competence.
It is the nursing profession's responsibility to shape and guide any process
for assuring nurse competence. Regulatory agencies define minimal standards of competence to protect the public. The employer is responsible and
accountable to provide a practice environment conducive to competent practice. Assurance of competence is the shared responsibility of the profession,
individual nurses, professional organizations, credentialing and certification
entities, regulatory agencies, employers, and other key stakeholders (ANA,
2014).

ANA believes that in the practice of nursing, competence can be defined,
measured, and evaluated. No single evaluation method or tool can guarantee

competence. Competence is situational and dynamic; it is both an outcome and an ongoing process. Context determines what competencies are necessary.

A number of terms and concepts are central to the discussion of the ongoing demonstration of competence:

> An individual who demonstrates competence is performing at an expected level.

- A *competency* is an expected level of performance that integrates knowledge, skills, abilities, and judgment.

- The integration of knowledge, skills, abilities, and judgment occurs in formal, informal, and reflective learning experiences.

- Knowledge encompasses thinking, understanding of science and humanities, professional standards of practice, and insights gained from context, practical experiences, personal capabilities, and leadership performance.

- Skills include psychomotor, communication, interpersonal, and diagnostic skills.

- Ability is the capacity to act effectively. It requires listening, integrity, knowledge of one's strengths and weaknesses, positive self-regard, emotional intelligence, and openness to feedback.

- Judgment includes critical thinking, problem solving, ethical reasoning, and decision-making. (ANA, 2014d, pp. 3–4)

When describing the types of learning associated with development of a competency, formal learning most often occurs in structured, academic, and professional development practice environments, while informal learning can be described as experiential insights gained in work, community, home, and other settings. The recurrent, thoughtful, personal self-assessment, analysis, and synthesis of strengths and opportunities for improvement constitute reflective learning. Such insights should lead to the creation of a specific plan for professional development and may become part of one's professional portfolio.

Competent registered nurses can be influenced by the nature of the situation, which includes consideration of the setting, resources, and the person. Situations can either enhance or detract from the nurse's ability to perform. The registered nurse influences factors that facilitate and enhance competent practice. Similarly, the nurse seeks to deal with barriers that constrain competent practice. The expected level of performance reflects variability depending upon context and the selected competence framework or model.

The ability to perform at the expected level requires a process of lifelong learning. Registered nurses must continually reassess their competencies and identify needs for additional knowledge, skills, personal growth, and integrative learning experiences.

Evaluating Competence

Competence in nursing practice can be evaluated by the individual nurse (self-assessment), nurse peers, and nurses in the roles of supervisor, coach, mentor, or preceptor. In addition, other aspects of nursing performance may be evaluated by professional colleagues and healthcare consumers.

Evaluation of competence involves the use of tools to capture objective and subjective data about the individual's knowledge base and actual performance. Those tools must be appropriate for the specific situation and the desired outcome of the competence evaluation. "However, no single evaluation tool or method can guarantee competence" (ANA, 2014d, p. 6).

Ongoing discussions and research on the definitions, meaning, evaluation, and relationship of competence and competency in educational and organizational literature inform nursing professionals about these topics (Hodges, 2010; Levine & Johnson, 2014). ANA supports this important work in the definition, measurement, and validation of nursing and healthcare professional competencies and values such major contributions as work associated with:

- Evidence-based nursing (Melnyk, Gallagher-Ford, Long, & Fineout-Overholt, 2014)

- Interprofessional competencies (IECEP, 2011)

- Leadership competencies (ANA, 2013c)

- Cultural competencies (Guidelines for Implementing Culturally Competent Nursing Care)

Professional Trends and Issues

Despite spending more on health care than any other nation, the United States ranks 23 out of 30 industrialized countries in life expectancy (Organization for Economic Cooperation and Development, 2014). A reformed healthcare system focused on primary care and prevention, quality and performance improvement initiatives (Weston & Roberts, 2013); interdisciplinary communication/collaboration; chronic disease management; and a healthy work environment for nurses and patients (ANA, 2015; U.S. Congress, 2013) can alleviate the financial and social costs of treating preventable and chronic diseases, improve patient and staff safety, and enhance nurse satisfaction and retention. Interprofessional teams, coordination of care across the illness trajectory, and technological advances will be key components in the new system—arenas in which nurses are familiar and have demonstrated their value.

Nurses at all levels are positioned to play key roles in a reformed and restructured care delivery system, such as:

- Coordinating healthcare consumers' transitions between healthcare delivery systems and settings (e.g., from hospital to rehabilitation to home);

- Assisting healthcare consumers monitor and manage wellness, acute illness, and chronic disease;

- Promoting integrative health and wellness;

- Providing preventive health care;

- Providing individualized care in nurse-managed health centers;

- Promoting enhanced data-driven decision-making;

- Participating in the "medical home" ("healthcare home") model for care management;

- Developing an expanded global health nursing perspective and platform;

- Operating as full partners, with physicians and other healthcare professionals, in redesigning health care in the United States (IOM, 2010);

- Assuring patient safety and quality are a part of nursing education (RWJF, 2011; IOM, 2010);

- Advancing APRNs' scope of practice consistent with education, training, and competencies (IOM, 2010); and

- Advocating for seamless academic progression and nursing school accreditation improvement at the national level.

Creating a Sustainable Nursing Workforce

The nursing shortage projected for the future presents a significant challenge to nurses to fill their critical role in health care. The Bureau of Labor Statistics' Employment Projections (2013) predicts the RN workforce will need to increase 19% to 3.24 million by 2022, a total of 1.05 million RN job openings. There is some good news on the horizon. According to the Organization for Economic Cooperation and Development (OECD, 2014), by the end of 2014, over half of the states were considering expanding the clinical duties of nurses, physician assistants (PAs), pharmacists, and others. By October 2014, New Jersey, Pennsylvania, and Michigan produced bills to expand the roles of nurse practitioners. In 2015, the aging nursing workforce, coupled with aging baby boomers, plus millions of new enrollees into the Universal Healthcare will be the impetus for states to allow nurses, nurse practitioners, PAs, and pharmacists to do more (AACN, 2014; OECD, 2013). Over the next five years, the number of primary care nurse practitioners and physician assistants is expected to increase by 30% and 58% respectively (OECD, 2013).

Nursing Education

Healthcare consumer needs and the care environment are more complex in the 21st century. Nurses have to make more critical decisions; be adept at using a variety of sophisticated, life-saving technology and information management systems; coordinate care among a variety of professional and community agencies; help healthcare consumers manage chronic illnesses; lead change from within their organizations; and affect national policy. Consequently, nursing students need to develop a broader range of competencies in the areas of health policy and healthcare financing (including understanding health insurance), community and public health, leadership, quality improvement, information management, and systems thinking, as well as become excellent clinicians (IOM, 2011).

According to the IOM (2011), in order to meet this demand, nurses should achieve higher levels of education, while educational systems and other stakeholders should support seamless academic progression and include innovative ways for nursing students to achieve their degrees through online, virtual, simulated, and competency-based learning. Curricula design should adequately prepare entry-level nurses and center on optimal patient outcomes. Schools of nursing must also build their capacities to prepare more graduate-level students to assume roles in advanced practice, leadership, teaching, and research (IOM, 2011).

Nursing as a profession continues to face dilemmas in entry into practice, recognition of the autonomy of advanced practice, maintenance of competence, complexity of multistate licensure, and the appropriate educational credentials for licensure and professional certification. Registered nurses have a professional responsibility to maintain competence in their area of practice. Employers who provide opportunities for professional development and continuing education promote a positive practice environment in which nurses can maintain and enhance skills and competencies.

This is an exciting time of progress and evolution for interprofessional education. According to the AACN (2015), "interdisciplinary education is when two or more disciplines collaborate in the learning process with the goal of fostering interprofessional interactions that enhance the practice of each discipline." Students from differing professions learn what each brings to the healthcare team and how each needs to foster communication, collaboration, conflict resolution, and mutual respect before graduation and entry into practice.

Technological Advances

Technology can drive effectiveness and efficiency, provide convenience, extend care to populations with little access to transportation, and serve as a major influence on how nurses practice (Huston, 2013; OECD, 2013). Technology can provide data transparency and offer a better work environment for nurses when designed and implemented in a manner that supports nurses' work and work flow. Work environments include conventional locations—hospitals, clinics, and healthcare consumer homes—as well as virtual spaces such as online discussion groups, email, interactive video, and virtual interaction (Cipriano, 2009). Ideally, technology eliminates redundancy and duplication of documentation, reduces errors, eliminates interruptions for missing supplies, equipment, and medications, and eases access to data, thereby allowing the nurse more time with the patient (Cipriano, 2009). Perhaps one of the most daunting challenges for nurses will be to retain the human element in practice. Other challenges include balancing cost with benefits, the daunting task of training the nursing workforce with a plan for sustainment, and assuring ethical use of technology (Huston, 2013).

Population Focus: Redefining Health and Well-being for the Millennial Generation

Insurers and health systems are looking for creative ways to attract, engage, and retain the 80 million millennial healthcare consumers born between 1980 and 2000 who have been shaped by the internet revolution. The millennials harbor different definitions and values of health and well-being, and are prompting society to rethink how one works, socializes, and interacts with the world. In 2015, they will help propel a New Health Economy that advances beyond health care to support a broader market of good health and well-being. National retailers are expected to expand service offerings related to health and well-being; private health exchanges to offer more holistic employee experiences; and new mobile technologies to create communities of personalized, real-time support, and feedback (OECD, 2013).

Baby Boomers: Health and Chronic Illness

The U.S. healthcare industry is under tremendous pressure to cut healthcare expenses for this population who are the costliest of all patients (OECD, 2013). Nurses have always been at the forefront of innovative and holistic care and are key to safe and effective management of high-cost patients in lower-cost care settings. One way this is being done is by "hotspotting," also called "social accountable care organization." This is a collaborative approach that uses effective care coordination to steer complex patients to lower-cost care settings instead of emergency rooms and inpatient beds. Medical, behavioral, and economic needs are addressed under these models. Millions of dollars have been saved utilizing these approaches (OECD, 2013; RWJF, 2014).

Whatever the practice venue in the next decade, registered nurses will continue to partner with others to advance the nation's health through many initiatives, such as *Healthy People 2020.* Such partnerships truly reflect the definition of nursing and illustrate the essential features of contemporary nursing practice (ANA, 2010b):

- A caring relationship that facilitates health and healing
- Attention to the range of human experiences and responses to health, disease, and illness in the physical and social environments
- Integration of global and environmental perspectives into nursing assessment
- Integration of objective data with knowledge gained from an appreciation of the healthcare consumer's or group's subjective experience
- Application of scientific knowledge to diagnosis and treatment through the use of judgment and critical thinking
- Advancement of professional nursing knowledge through scholarly inquiry.
- Influence on social and public policy to promote social justice.

Summary of the Scope of Nursing Practice

The dynamic nature of the healthcare practice environment and the growing body of nursing research provide both the impetus and the opportunity for nursing to ensure competent nursing practice in all settings for all healthcare consumers, and to promote ongoing professional development that enhances the quality of nursing practice. *Nursing: Scope and Standards of Practice, Third Edition* assists that process by delineating the professional scope and standards of practice and responsibilities of all professional registered nurses in every setting. As such, this resource can serve as a basis for:

- Quality improvement systems
- Healthcare reimbursement and financing methodologies

- Development and evaluation of nursing service delivery systems and organizational structures
- Certification activities
- Position descriptions and performance appraisals
- Agency policies, procedures, and protocols
- Regulatory systems
- Educational offerings
- Establishing the legal standard of care

Standards of Professional Nursing Practice

Significance of Standards

The Standards of Professional Nursing Practice are authoritative statements of the duties that all registered nurses, regardless of role, population, or specialty, are expected to perform competently. The standards published herein may be utilized as evidence of the standard of care, with the understanding that application of the standards is context dependent. The standards are subject to change with the dynamics of the nursing profession, as new patterns of professional practice are developed and accepted by the nursing profession and the public. In addition, specific conditions and clinical circumstances may also affect the application of the standards at a given time (e.g., during a natural disaster). The standards are subject to formal, periodic review and revision.

The competencies that accompany each standard may be evidence of compliance with the corresponding standard. The list of competencies is not exhaustive. Whether a particular standard or competency applies depends upon the circumstances. The competencies are presented for the registered nurse level and are applicable for *all* nurses. Standards may include additional competencies delineated for the graduate-level prepared registered nurse, a category that also includes advanced practice registered nurses. In some instances, additional discrete competencies applicable only to advanced practice registered nurses may be included.

Standards of Practice

Standard 1. Assessment
The registered nurse collects pertinent data and information relative to the healthcare consumer's health or the situation.

Competencies
The registered nurse:

- ▶ Collects pertinent data, including but not limited to demographics, social determinants of health, health disparities, and physical, functional, psychosocial, emotional, cognitive, sexual, cultural, age-related, environmental, spiritual/transpersonal, and economic assessments in a systematic, ongoing process with compassion and respect for the inherent dignity, worth, and unique attributes of every person.

- ▶ Recognizes the importance of the assessment parameters identified by WHO (World Health Organization), *Healthy People 2020*, or other organizations that influence nursing practice.

- ▶ Integrates knowledge from global and environmental factors into the assessment process.

- ▶ Elicits the healthcare consumer's values, preferences, expressed and unexpressed needs, and knowledge of the healthcare situation.

- ▶ Recognizes the impact of one's own personal attitudes, values, and beliefs on the assessment process.

- ▶ Identifies barriers to effective communication based on psychosocial, literacy, financial, and cultural considerations.

- ▶ Assesses the impact of family dynamics on healthcare consumer health and wellness.

- Engages the healthcare consumer and other interprofessional team members in holistic, culturally sensitive data collection.

- Prioritizes data collection based on the healthcare consumer's immediate condition or the anticipated needs of the healthcare consumer or situation.

- Uses evidence-based assessment techniques, instruments, tools, available data, information, and knowledge relevant to the situation to identify patterns and variances.

- Applies ethical, legal, and privacy guidelines and policies to the collection, maintenance, use, and dissemination of data and information.

- Recognizes the healthcare consumer as the authority on their own health by honoring their care preferences.

- Documents relevant data accurately and in a manner accessible to the interprofessional team.

Additional competencies for the graduate-level prepared registered nurse

In addition to the registered nurse competencies, the graduate-level prepared registered nurse and the advanced practice registered nurse:

- Assesses the effect of interactions among individuals, family, community, and social systems on health and illness.

- Synthesizes the results and information leading to clinical understanding.

Additional competencies for the advanced practice registered nurse

In addition to the competencies of the registered nurse and the graduate-level prepared registered nurse, the advanced practice registered nurse:

- Initiates diagnostic tests and procedures relevant to the healthcare consumer's current status.

- Uses advanced assessment, knowledge, and skills to maintain, enhance, or improve health conditions.

Standard 2. Diagnosis
The registered nurse analyzes assessment data to determine actual or potential diagnoses, problems, and issues.

Competencies
The registered nurse:

> ▶ Identifies actual or potential risks to the healthcare consumer's health and safety or barriers to health, which may include but are not limited to interpersonal, systematic, cultural, or environmental circumstances.

> ▶ Uses assessment data, standardized classification systems, technology, and clinical decision support tools to articulate actual or potential diagnoses, problems, and issues.

> ▶ Verifies the diagnoses, problems, and issues with the individual, family, group, community, population, and interprofessional colleagues.

> ▶ Prioritizes diagnoses, problems, and issues based on mutually established goals to meet the needs of the healthcare consumer across the health–illness continuum.

> ▶ Documents diagnoses, problems, and issues in a manner that facilitates the determination of the expected outcomes and plan.

Additional competencies for the graduate-level prepared registered nurse
In addition to the competencies of the registered nurse, the graduate-level prepared registered nurse:

> ▶ Uses information and communication technologies to analyze diagnostic practice patterns of nurses and other members of the interprofessional healthcare team.

> ▶ Employs aggregate-level data to articulate diagnoses, problems, and issues of healthcare consumers and organizational systems.

Additional competencies for the advanced practice registered nurse

In addition to the competencies of the registered nurse and the graduate-level prepared registered nurse, the advanced practice registered nurse:

▶ Formulates a differential diagnosis based on the assessment, history, physical examination, and diagnostic test results.

Standard 3. Outcomes Identification

The registered nurse identifies expected outcomes for a plan individualized to the healthcare consumer or the situation.

Competencies

The registered nurse:

- ▶ Engages the healthcare consumer, interprofessional team, and others in partnership to identify expected outcomes.

- ▶ Formulates culturally sensitive expected outcomes derived from assessments and diagnoses.

- ▶ Uses clinical expertise and current evidence-based practice to identify health risks, benefits, costs, and/or expected trajectory of the condition.

- ▶ Collaborates with the healthcare consumer to define expected outcomes integrating the healthcare consumer's culture, values, and ethical considerations.

- ▶ Generates a time frame for the attainment of expected outcomes.

- ▶ Develops expected outcomes that facilitate coordination of care.

- ▶ Modifies expected outcomes based on the evaluation of the status of the healthcare consumer and situation.

- ▶ Documents expected outcomes as measurable goals.

- ▶ Evaluates the actual outcomes in relation to expected outcomes, safety, and quality standards.

Additional competencies for the graduate-level prepared registered nurse, including the APRN

In addition to the competencies of the registered nurse, the graduate-level prepared registered nurse or advanced practice registered nurse:

- ▶ Defines expected outcomes that incorporate cost, clinical effectiveness, and are aligned with the outcomes identified by members of the interprofessional team.

- ▶ Differentiates outcomes that require care process interventions from those that require system-level actions.

- ▶ Integrates scientific evidence and best practices to achieve expected outcomes.

► Advocates for outcomes that reflect the healthcare consumer's culture, values, and ethical concerns.

Standard 4. Planning
The registered nurse develops a plan that prescribes strategies to attain expected, measurable outcomes.

Competencies
The registered nurse:

▶ Develops an individualized, holistic, evidence-based plan in partnership with the healthcare consumer and interprofessional team.

▶ Establishes the plan priorities with the healthcare consumer and interprofessional team.

▶ Advocates for responsible and appropriate use of interventions to minimize unwarranted or unwanted treatment and/or healthcare consumer suffering.

▶ Prioritizes elements of the plan based on the assessment of the healthcare consumer's level of risk and safety needs.

▶ Includes evidence-based strategies in the plan to address each of the identified diagnoses, problems, or issues. These strategies may include but are not limited to:

  ▶ Promotion and restoration of health,

  ▶ Prevention of illness, injury, and disease,

  ▶ Facilitation of healing,

  ▶ Alleviation of suffering, and

  ▶ Supportive care

▶ Incorporates an implementation pathway that describes steps and milestones.

▶ Identifies cost and economic implications of the plan.

▶ Develops a plan that reflects compliance with current statutes, rules and regulations, and standards.

▶ Modifies the plan according to the ongoing assessment of the healthcare consumer's response and other outcome indicators.

▶ Documents the plan using standardized language or recognized terminology.

Additional competencies for the graduate-level prepared registered nurse

In addition to the competencies of the registered nurse, the graduate-level prepared registered nurse:

> ▶ Designs strategies and tactics to meet the multifaceted and complex needs of healthcare consumers or others.

> ▶ Leads the design and development of interprofessional processes to address the identified diagnoses, problems, or issues.

> ▶ Designs innovative nursing practices.

> ▶ Actively participates in the development and continuous improvement of systems that support the planning process.

Additional competencies for the advanced practice registered nurse

In addition to the competencies of the registered nurse and graduate-level prepared registered nurse, the advanced practice registered nurse:

> ▶ Integrates assessment strategies, diagnostic strategies, and therapeutic interventions that reflect current evidence-based knowledge and practice.

Standard 5. Implementation

The registered nurse implements the identified plan.

Competencies

The registered nurse:

- ▶ Partners with the healthcare consumer to implement the plan in a safe, effective, efficient, timely, patient-centered, and equitable manner (IOM, 2010).

- ▶ Integrates interprofessional team partners in implementation of the plan through collaboration and communication across the continuum of care.

- ▶ Demonstrates caring behaviors to develop therapeutic relationships.

- ▶ Provides culturally congruent, holistic care that focuses on the healthcare consumer and addresses and advocates for the needs of diverse populations across the lifespan.

- ▶ Uses evidence-based interventions and strategies to achieve the mutually identified goals and outcomes specific to the problem or needs.

- ▶ Integrates critical thinking and technology solutions to implement the nursing process to collect, measure, record, retrieve, trend, and analyze data and information to enhance nursing practice and healthcare consumer outcomes.

- ▶ Delegates according to the health, safety, and welfare of the healthcare consumer and considering the circumstance, person, task, direction or communication, supervision, evaluation, as well as the state nurse practice act regulations, institution, and regulatory entities while maintaining accountability for the care.

- ▶ Documents implementation and any modifications, including changes or omissions, of the identified plan.

Additional competencies for the graduate-level prepared registered nurse

In addition to the competencies of the registered nurse, the graduate-level prepared registered nurse:

- ▶ Uses systems, organizations, and community resources to lead effective change and implement the plan.

- Applies quality principles while articulating methods, tools, performance measures, and standards as they relate to implementation of the plan.

- Translates evidence into practice.

- Leads interprofessional teams to communicate, collaborate, and consult effectively.

- Demonstrates leadership skills that emphasize ethical and critical decision-making, effective working relationships, and a systems perspective.

- Serves as a consultant to provide additional insight and potential solutions.

- Uses theory-driven approaches to effect organizational or system change.

Additional competencies for the advanced practice registered nurse

In addition to the competencies of the registered nurse and graduate-level prepared registered nurse, the advanced practice registered nurse:

- Uses prescriptive authority, procedures, referrals, treatments, and therapies in accordance with state and federal laws and regulations.

- Prescribes traditional and integrative evidence-based treatments, therapies, and procedures that are compatible with the healthcare consumer's cultural preferences and norms.

- Prescribes evidence-based pharmacological agents and treatments according to clinical indicators and results of diagnostic and laboratory tests.

- Provides clinical consultation for healthcare consumers and professionals related to complex clinical cases to improve care and patient outcomes.

Standard 5A. Coordination of Care

The registered nurse coordinates care delivery.

Competencies

The registered nurse:

- ▶ Organizes the components of the plan.

- ▶ Collaborates with the consumer to help manage health care based on mutually agreed upon outcomes.

- ▶ Manages a healthcare consumer's care in order to reach mutually agreed upon outcomes.

- ▶ Engages healthcare consumers in self-care to achieve preferred goals for quality of life.

- ▶ Assists the healthcare consumer to identify options for care.

- ▶ Communicates with the healthcare consumer, interprofessional team, and community-based resources to effect safe transitions in continuity of care.

- ▶ Advocates for the delivery of dignified and holistic care by the interprofessional team.

- ▶ Documents the coordination of care.

Additional competencies for the graduate-level prepared registered nurse

In addition to the competencies of the registered nurse, the graduate-level prepared registered nurse:

- ▶ Provides leadership in the coordination of interprofessional health care for integrated delivery of healthcare consumer services to achieve safe, effective, efficient, timely, patient-centered, and equitable care (IOM, 2010).

Additional competencies for the advanced practice registered nurse

In addition to the competencies of the registered nurse and graduate-level prepared registered nurse, the advanced practice registered nurse:

▶ Manages identified consumer panels or populations.

▶ Serves as the healthcare consumer's primary care provider and coordinator of healthcare services in accordance with state and federal laws and regulations.

▶ Synthesizes data and information to prescribe and provide necessary system and community support measures, including modifications of environments.

Standard 5B. Health Teaching and Health Promotion

The registered nurse employs strategies to promote health and a safe environment.

Competencies

The registered nurse:

- ▶ Provides opportunities for the healthcare consumer to identify needed healthcare promotion, disease prevention, and self-management topics.

- ▶ Uses health promotion and health teaching methods in collaboration with the healthcare consumer's values, beliefs, health practices, developmental level, learning needs, readiness and ability to learn, language preference, spirituality, culture, and socioeconomic status.

- ▶ Uses feedback and evaluations from the healthcare consumer to determine the effectiveness of the employed strategies.

- ▶ Uses technologies to communicate health promotion and disease prevention information to the healthcare consumer.

- ▶ Provides healthcare consumers with information about intended effects and potential adverse effects of the plan of care.

- ▶ Engages consumer alliance and advocacy groups in health teaching and health promotion activities for healthcare consumers.

- ▶ Provides anticipatory guidance to healthcare consumers to promote health and prevent or reduce the risk of negative health outcomes.

Additional competencies for the graduate-level prepared registered nurse, including the APRN

In addition to the competencies of the registered nurse, the graduate-level prepared registered nurse or advanced practice registered nurse:

- ▶ Synthesizes empirical evidence on risk behaviors, gender roles, learning theories, behavioral change theories, motivational theories, translational theories for evidence-based practice, epidemiology, and other related theories and frameworks when designing health education information and programs.

- ▶ Evaluates health information resources for applicability, accuracy, readability, and comprehensibility to help healthcare consumers access quality health information.

Standard 6. Evaluation

The registered nurse evaluates progress toward attainment of goals and outcomes.

Competencies

The registered nurse:

▶ Conducts a holistic, systematic, ongoing, and criterion-based evaluation of the goals and outcomes in relation to the structure, processes, and timeline prescribed in the plan.

▶ Collaborates with the healthcare consumer and others involved in the care or situation in the evaluation process.

▶ Determines, in partnership with the healthcare consumer and other stakeholders, the patient-centeredness, effectiveness, efficiency, safety, timeliness, and equitability (IOM, 2001) of the strategies in relation to the responses to the plan and attainment of outcomes. Other defined criteria (e.g., Quality and Safety Education for Nurses) may be used as well.

▶ Uses ongoing assessment data to revise the diagnoses, outcomes, plan, and implementation strategies.

▶ Shares evaluation data and conclusions with the healthcare consumer and other stakeholders in accordance with federal and state regulations.

▶ Documents the results of the evaluation.

Additional competencies for the graduate-level prepared registered nurse, including the APRN

In addition to the competencies of the registered nurse, the graduate-level prepared registered nurse or the advanced practice registered nurse:

▶ Synthesizes evaluation data from the healthcare consumer, community, population and/or institution to determine the effectiveness of the plan.

▶ Engages in a systematic evaluation process to revise the plan to enhance its effectiveness.

▶ Uses results of the evaluation to make or recommend process, policy, procedure, or protocol revisions when warranted.

Standards of Professional Performance

Standard 7. Ethics
The registered nurse practices ethically.

Competencies
The registered nurse:

- ▶ Integrates the *Code of Ethics for Nurses with Interpretive Statements* (ANA, 2015) to guide nursing practice and articulate the moral foundation of nursing.

- ▶ Practices with compassion and respect for the inherent dignity, worth, and unique attributes of all people.

- ▶ Advocates for healthcare consumers' rights to informed decision-making and self-determination.

- ▶ Seeks guidance in situations where the rights of the individual conflict with public health guidelines.

- ▶ Endorses the understanding that the primary commitment is to the healthcare consumer regardless of setting or situation.

- ▶ Maintains therapeutic relationships and professional boundaries.

- ▶ Advocates for the rights, health, and safety of the healthcare consumer and others.

- ▶ Safeguards the privacy and confidentiality of healthcare consumers, others, and their data and information within ethical, legal, and regulatory parameters.

- ▶ Demonstrates professional accountability and responsibility for nursing practice.

- ▶ Maintains competence through continued personal and professional development.

- ▶ Demonstrates commitment to self-reflection and self-care.

- ▶ Contributes to the establishment and maintenance of an ethical environment that is conducive to safe, quality health care.

- ▶ Advances the profession through scholarly inquiry, professional standards development, and the generation of policy.

- ▶ Collaborates with other health professionals and the public to protect human rights, promote health diplomacy, enhance cultural sensitivity and congruence, and reduce health disparities.

- ▶ Articulates nursing values to maintain personal integrity and the integrity of the profession.

- ▶ Integrates principles of social justice into nursing and policy.

Standard 8. Culturally Congruent Practice

The registered nurse practices in a manner that is congruent with cultural diversity and inclusion principles.

Competencies

The registered nurse:

▶ Demonstrates respect, equity, and empathy in actions and interactions with all healthcare consumers.

▶ Participates in life-long learning to understand cultural preferences, worldview, choices, and decision-making processes of diverse consumers.

▶ Creates an inventory of one's own values, beliefs, and cultural heritage.

▶ Applies knowledge of variations in health beliefs, practices, and communication patterns in all nursing practice activities.

▶ Identifies the stage of the consumer's acculturation and accompanying patterns of needs and engagement.

▶ Considers the effects and impact of discrimination and oppression on practice within and among vulnerable cultural groups.

▶ Uses skills and tools that are appropriately vetted for the culture, literacy, and language of the population served.

▶ Communicates with appropriate language and behaviors, including the use of medical interpreters and translators in accordance with consumer preferences.

▶ Identifies the cultural-specific meaning of interactions, terms, and content.

▶ Respects consumer decisions based on age, tradition, belief and family influence, and stage of acculturation.

▶ Advocates for policies that promote health and prevent harm among culturally diverse, under-served, or under-represented consumers.

▶ Promotes equal access to services, tests, interventions, health promotion programs, enrollment in research, education, and other opportunities.

> Educates nurse colleagues and other professionals about cultural similarities and differences of healthcare consumers, families, groups, communities, and populations.

Additional competencies for the graduate-level prepared registered nurse

In addition to the competencies of the registered nurse, the graduate-level prepared registered nurse:

> Evaluates tools, instruments, and services provided to culturally diverse populations.

> Advances organizational policies, programs, services, and practice that reflect respect, equity, and values for diversity and inclusion.

> Engages consumers, key stakeholders, and others in designing and establishing internal and external cross-cultural partnerships.

> Conducts research to improve health care and healthcare outcomes for culturally diverse consumers.

> Develops recruitment and retention strategies to achieve a multicultural workforce.

Additional competencies for the advanced practice registered nurse

In addition to the competencies of the registered nurse and graduate-level prepared registered nurse, the advanced practice registered nurse:

> Promotes shared decision-making solutions in planning, prescribing, and evaluating processes when the healthcare consumer's cultural preferences and norms may create incompatibility with evidence-based practice.

> Leads interprofessional teams to identify the cultural and language needs of the consumer.

Standard 9. Communication

The registered nurse communicates effectively in all areas of practice.

Competencies

The registered nurse:

- ▶ Assesses one's own communication skills and effectiveness.

- ▶ Demonstrates cultural empathy when communicating.

- ▶ Assesses communication ability, health literacy, resources, and preferences of healthcare consumers to inform the interprofessional team and others.

- ▶ Uses language translation resources to ensure effective communication.

- ▶ Incorporates appropriate alternative strategies to communicate effectively with healthcare consumers who have visual, speech, language, or communication difficulties.

- ▶ Uses communication styles and methods that demonstrate caring, respect, deep listening, authenticity, and trust.

- ▶ Conveys accurate information.

- ▶ Maintains communication with interprofessional team and others to facilitate safe transitions and continuity in care delivery.

- ▶ Contributes the nursing perspective in interactions with others and discussions with the interprofessional team.

- ▶ Exposes care processes and decisions when they do not appear to be in the best interest of the healthcare consumer.

- ▶ Discloses concerns related to potential or actual hazards and errors in care or the practice environment to the appropriate level.

- ▶ Demonstrates continuous improvement of communication skills.

Additional competencies for the graduate-level prepared registered nurse, including the APRN

In addition to the competencies of the registered nurse, the graduate-level prepared registered nurse or advanced practice registered nurse:

▶ Assumes a leadership role in shaping or fashioning environments that promote healthy communication.

Standard 10. Collaboration
The registered nurse collaborates with the healthcare consumer and other key stakeholders in the conduct of nursing practice.

Competencies
The registered nurse:

- Identifies the areas of expertise and contribution of other professionals and key stakeholders.
- Clearly articulates the nurse's role and responsibilities within the team.
- Uses the unique and complementary abilities of all members of the team to optimize attainment of desired outcomes.
- Partners with the healthcare consumer and key stakeholders to advocate for and effect change, leading to positive outcomes and quality care.
- Uses appropriate tools and techniques, including information systems and technologies, to facilitate discussion and team functions, in a manner that protects dignity, respect, privacy, and confidentiality.
- Promotes engagement through consensus building and conflict management.
- Uses effective group dynamics and strategies to enhance team performance.
- Exhibits dignity and respect when interacting with others and giving and receiving feedback.
- Partners with all stakeholders to create, implement, and evaluate a comprehensive plan.

Additional competencies for the graduate-level prepared registered nurse, including the APRN
In addition to the competencies of the registered nurse, the graduate-level prepared registered nurse, or advanced practice registered nurse:

- Participates in interprofessional activities, including but not limited to education, consultation, management, technological development, or research to enhance outcomes.

▶ Provides leadership for establishing, improving, and sustaining collaborative relationships to achieve safe, quality care for healthcare consumers.

▶ Advances interprofessional plan-of-care documentation and communications, rationales for plan-of-care changes, and collaborative discussions to improve healthcare consumer outcomes.

Standard 11. Leadership
The registered nurse leads within the professional practice setting and the profession.

Competencies
The registered nurse:

▶ Contributes to the establishment of an environment that supports and maintains respect, trust, and dignity.

▶ Encourages innovation in practice and role performance to attain personal and professional plans, goals, and vision.

▶ Communicates to manage change and address conflict.

▶ Mentors colleagues for the advancement of nursing practice and the profession to enhance safe, quality health care.

▶ Retains accountability for delegated nursing care.

▶ Contributes to the evolution of the profession through participation in professional organizations.

▶ Influences policy to promote health.

Additional competencies for the graduate-level prepared registered nurse, including the APRN
In addition to the competencies of the registered nurse, the graduate-level prepared registered nurse or advanced practice registered nurse:

▶ Influences decision-making bodies to improve the professional practice environment and healthcare consumer outcomes.

▶ Enhances the effectiveness of the interprofessional team.

▶ Promotes advanced practice nursing and role development by interpreting its role for healthcare consumers and policy makers.

▶ Models expert practice to interprofessional team members and healthcare consumers.

▶ Mentors colleagues in the acquisition of clinical knowledge, skills, abilities, and judgment.

Standard 12. Education

The registered nurse seeks knowledge and competence that reflects current nursing practice and promotes futuristic thinking.

Competencies

The registered nurse:

▶ Identifies learning needs based on nursing knowledge and the various roles the nurse may assume.

▶ Participates in ongoing educational activities related to nursing and interprofessional knowledge bases and professional topics.

▶ Mentors nurses new to their roles for the purpose of ensuring successful enculturation, orientation, and emotional support.

▶ Demonstrates a commitment to lifelong learning through self-reflection and inquiry for learning and personal growth.

▶ Seeks experiences that reflect current practice to maintain and advance knowledge, skills, abilities, attitudes, and judgment in clinical practice or role performance.

▶ Acquires knowledge and skills relative to the role, population, specialty, setting, and global or local health situation.

▶ Participates in formal consultations or informal discussions to address issues in nursing practice as an application of education and knowledge.

▶ Identifies modifications or accommodations needed in the delivery of education based on healthcare consumer and family members' needs.

▶ Shares educational findings, experiences, and ideas with peers.

▶ Supports acculturation of nurses new to their roles by role modeling, encouraging, and sharing pertinent information relative to optimal care delivery.

▶ Facilitates a work environment supportive of ongoing education of healthcare professionals.

▶ Maintains a professional portfolio that provides evidence of individual competence and lifelong learning.

Standard 13. Evidence-based Practice and Research
The registered nurse integrates evidence and research findings into practice.

Competencies
The registered nurse:

- ▶ Articulates the values of research and its application relative to the healthcare setting and practice.

- ▶ Identifies questions in the healthcare setting and practice that can be answered by nursing research.

- ▶ Uses current evidence-based knowledge, including research findings, to guide practice.

- ▶ Incorporates evidence when initiating changes in nursing practice.

- ▶ Participates in the formulation of evidence-based practice through research.

- ▶ Promotes ethical principles of research in practice and the health-care setting.

- ▶ Appraises nursing research for optimal application in practice and the healthcare setting.

- ▶ Shares peer reviewed research findings with colleagues to integrate knowledge into nursing practice.

Additional competencies for the graduate-level prepared registered nurse, including the APRN
In addition to the competencies of the registered nurse, the graduate-level prepared registered nurse or advanced practice registered nurse:

- ▶ Integrates research-based practice in all settings.

- ▶ Uses current healthcare research findings and other evidence to expand knowledge, skills, abilities, and judgment; to enhance role performance; and to increase knowledge of professional issues.

- ▶ Uses critical thinking skills to connect theory and research to practice.

- ▶ Integrates nursing research to improve quality in nursing practice.

▶ Contributes to nursing knowledge by conducting or synthesizing research and other evidence that discovers, examines, and evaluates current practice, knowledge, theories, criteria, and creative approaches to improve healthcare outcomes.

▶ Encourages other nurses to develop research skills.

▶ Performs rigorous critique of evidence derived from databases to generate meaningful evidence for nursing practice.

▶ Advocates for the ethical conduct of research and translational scholarship with particular attention to the protection of the healthcare consumer as a research participant.

▶ Promotes a climate of collaborative research and clinical inquiry.

▶ Disseminates research findings through activities such as presentations, publications, consultation, and journal clubs.

Standard 14. Quality of Practice
The registered nurse contributes to quality nursing practice.

Competencies
The registered nurse:

▶ Ensures that nursing practice is safe, effective, efficient, equitable, timely, and patient-centered (IOM, 1999; IOM, 2001).

▶ Identifies barriers and opportunities to improve healthcare safety, effectiveness, efficiency, equitability, timeliness, and patient-centeredness.

▶ Recommends strategies to improve nursing quality.

▶ Uses creativity and innovation to enhance nursing care.

▶ Participates in quality improvement initiatives.

▶ Collects data to monitor the quality of nursing practice.

▶ Contributes in efforts to improve healthcare efficiency.

▶ Provides critical review and/or evaluation of policies, procedures, and guidelines to improve the quality of health care.

▶ Engages in formal and informal peer review processes.

▶ Collaborates with the interprofessional team to implement quality improvement plans and interventions.

▶ Documents nursing practice in a manner that supports quality and performance improvement initiatives.

▶ Achieves professional certification, when available.

Additional competencies for the graduate-level prepared registered nurse
In addition to the competencies for the registered nurse, the graduate-level prepared registered nurse:

▶ Analyzes trends in healthcare quality data, including examination of cultural influences and factors.

▶ Incorporates evidence into nursing practice to improve outcomes.

▶ Designs innovations to improve outcomes.

- Provides leadership in the design and implementation of quality improvement initiatives.

- Promotes a practice environment that supports evidence-based health care.

- Contributes to nursing and interprofessional knowledge through scientific inquiry.

- Encourages professional or specialty certification.

- Engages in development, implementation, evaluation, and/or revision of policies, procedures, and guidelines to improve healthcare quality.

- Uses data and information in system-level decision-making.

- Influences the organizational system to improve outcomes.

Additional competencies for the advanced practice registered nurse

In addition to the competencies for the registered nurse and graduate-level prepared registered nurse, the advanced practice registered nurse:

- Engages in comparison evaluations of the effectiveness and efficacy of diagnostic tests, clinical procedures and therapies, and treatment plans, in partnership with healthcare consumers, to optimize health and healthcare quality.

- Designs quality improvement studies, research, initiatives, and programs to improve health outcomes in diverse settings.

- Applies knowledge obtained from advanced preparation, as well as current research and evidence-based information, to clinical decision-making at the point of care to achieve optimal health outcomes.

- Uses available benchmarks as a means to evaluate practice at the individual, departmental, or organizational level.

Standard 15. Professional Practice Evaluation
The registered nurse evaluates one's own and others' nursing practice.

Competencies
The registered nurse:

► Engages in self-reflection and self-evaluation of nursing practice on a regular basis, identifying areas of strength as well as areas in which professional growth would be beneficial.

► Adheres to the guidance about professional practice as specified in the *Nursing: Scope and Standards of Practice* and the *Code of Ethics for Nurses with Interpretive Statements*.

► Ensures that nursing practice is consistent with regulatory requirements pertaining to licensure, relevant statutes, rules, and regulations.

► Uses organizational policies and procedures to guide professional practice.

► Influences organizational policies and procedures to promote inter-professional evidence-based practice.

► Provides evidence for practice decisions and actions as part of the formal and informal evaluation processes.

► Seeks formal and informal feedback regarding one's own practice from healthcare consumers, peers, colleagues, supervisors, and others.

► Provides peers and others with formal and informal constructive feedback regarding their practice or role performance.

► Takes action to achieve goals identified during the evaluation process.

Standard 16. Resource Utilization

The registered nurse utilizes appropriate resources to plan, provide, and sustain evidence-based nursing services that are safe, effective, and fiscally responsible.

Competencies

The registered nurse:

- ▶ Assesses healthcare consumer care needs and resources available to achieve desired outcomes.

- ▶ Assists the healthcare consumer in factoring costs, risks, and benefits in decisions about care.

- ▶ Assists the healthcare consumer in identifying and securing appropriate services to address needs across the healthcare continuum.

- ▶ Delegates in accordance with applicable legal and policy parameters.

- ▶ Identifies impact of resource allocation on the potential for harm, complexity of the task, and desired outcomes.

- ▶ Advocates for resources that support and enhance nursing practice.

- ▶ Integrates telehealth and mobile health technologies into practice to promote positive interactions between healthcare consumers and care providers.

- ▶ Uses organizational and community resources to implement interprofessional plans.

- ▶ Addresses discriminatory healthcare practices and the impact on resource allocation.

Additional competencies for the graduate-level prepared registered nurse

In addition to the competencies of the registered nurse, the graduate-level prepared registered nurse:

- ▶ Designs innovative solutions to use resources effectively and maintain quality.

- ▶ Creates evaluation strategies that address cost effectiveness, cost benefit, and efficiency factors associated with nursing practice.

- ▶ Assumes complex and advanced leadership roles to initiate and guide change.

Additional competencies for the advanced practice registered nurse

In addition to the competencies of the registered nurse and graduate-level prepared registered nurse, the advanced practice registered nurse:

▶ Engages organizational and community resources to formulate and implement interprofessional plans.

Standard 17. Environmental Health

The registered nurse practices in an environmentally safe and healthy manner.

Competencies

The registered nurse:

▶ Promotes a safe and healthy workplace and professional practice environment.

▶ Uses environmental health concepts in practice.

▶ Assesses the environment to identify risk factors.

▶ Reduces environmental health risks to self, colleagues, and health-care consumers.

▶ Communicates information about environmental health risks and exposure reduction strategies.

▶ Advocates for the safe, judicious, and appropriate use and disposal of products in health care.

▶ Incorporates technologies to promote safe practice environments.

▶ Uses products or treatments consistent with evidence-based practice to reduce environmental threats.

▶ Participates in developing strategies to promote healthy communities and practice environments.

Additional competencies for the graduate-level prepared registered nurse, including the APRN

In addition to the competencies of the registered nurse, the graduate-level prepared registered nurse:

▶ Analyzes the impact of social, political, and economic influences on the global environment and human health experience.

▶ Creates partnerships that promote sustainable global environmental health policies and conditions that focus on prevention of hazards to people and the natural environment (ANA, 2007).

Glossary

Acculturation.   The process by which an individual or group from one culture learns how to take on many of the behaviors, values, and ways of living of another culture. Few cultures become 100% acculturated to another cultural way of life. Cultures tend to be selective in what they choose to change and retain (Leininger, 1995, pp. 72–73).

Advanced practice registered nurse (APRN).   A registered nurse who has completed an accredited graduate-level education program preparing her or him for the role of certified nurse practitioner, certified registered nurse anesthetist, certified nurse midwife, or clinical nurse specialist; has passed a national certification examination that measures the APRN role and population-focused competencies; maintains continued competence as evidenced by recertification; and is licensed to practice as an APRN. (See 2008 APRN Consensus Model for detailed definition.)

Assessment.   A systematic, dynamic process by which the registered nurse, through interaction with the patient, family, groups, communities, populations, and healthcare providers, collects and analyzes data. Assessment may include the following dimensions: physical, psychological, socio-cultural, spiritual, cognitive, functional abilities, developmental, economic, and lifestyle.

Autonomy.   The capacity of a nurse to determine her or his own actions through independent choice, including demonstration of competence, within the full scope of nursing practice.

Caring.   The moral ideal of nursing consisting of human-to-human attempts to protect, enhance, and preserve humanity and human dignity, integrity, and wholeness by assisting a person to find meaning in illness, suffering, pain, and existence (Watson, 2012).

Caregiver.   A person who provides direct care for another, such as a child, dependent adult, the disabled, or the chronically ill.

Code of ethics (nursing). A list of provisions that makes explicit the primary goals, values, and obligations of the nursing profession and expresses its values, duties, and commitments to the society of which it is a part. In the United States, nurses abide by and adhere to *Code of Ethics for Nurses with Interpretive Statements* (ANA, 2015).

Collaboration. A professional healthcare partnership grounded in a reciprocal and respectful recognition and acceptance of: each partner's unique expertise, power, and sphere of influence and responsibilities; the commonality of goals; the mutual safeguarding of the legitimate interest of each party; and the advantages of such a relationship.

Competency. An expected and measureable level of nursing performance that integrates knowledge, skills, abilities, and judgment, based on established scientific knowledge and expectations for nursing practice.

Continuity of care. An interprofessional process that includes healthcare consumers, families, and other stakeholders in the development of a coordinated plan of care. This process facilitates the patient's transition between settings and healthcare providers, based on changing needs and available resources.

Cultural knowledge. The concepts and language of an ethnic or social group used to describe their health-related values, beliefs, and traditional practices, as well as the etiologies of their conditions, preferred treatments, and any contraindications for treatments or pharmacological interventions. Historical events, such as war-related migration, oppression, and structural discrimination are also included, when relevant.

Cultural skills. The integration of cultural knowledge and expertise into practice when assessing, communicating with, and providing care for members of a racial, ethnic or social group.

Delegation. The transfer of responsibility for the performance of a task from one individual to another while retaining accountability for the outcome. Example: The RN, in delegating a task to an assistive individual, transfers the responsibility for the performance of the task but retains professional accountability for the overall care.

Diagnosis. A clinical judgment about the healthcare consumers' response to actual or potential health conditions or needs. The diagnosis provides the basis for determination of a plan to achieve expected outcomes. Registered nurses utilize nursing and medical diagnoses depending upon educational and clinical preparation and legal authority.

Ecosystem. A system, or a group of interconnected elements, formed by the interaction of a community of organisms with their environment.

Environment. The surrounding habitat, context, milieu, conditions, and atmosphere in which all living systems participate and interact. It includes the physical habitat as well as cultural, psychological, social, and historical influences. It includes both the external physical space as well as an individual's internal physical, mental, emotional, social, and spiritual experience (ANA & AHNA, 2013)

Environmental health. Aspects of human health, including quality of life, that are determined by physical, chemical, biological, social, and psychological influences in the environment. It also refers to the theory and practice of assessing, correcting, controlling, and preventing those factors in the environment that can potentially adversely affect the health of present and future generations.

Evaluation. The process of determining the progress toward attainment of expected outcomes, including the effectiveness of care.

Evidence-based practice. A life-long problem-solving approach that integrates the best evidence from well-designed research studies and evidence-based theories; clinical expertise and evidence from assessment of the health consumer's history and condition, as well as healthcare resources; and patient, family, group, community, and population preferences and values. When EBP is delivered in a context of caring, as well as an ecosystem or environment that supports it, the best clinical decisions are made to yield positive healthcare consumer outcomes (Melnyk, Gallagher-Ford, Long, & Fineout-Overholt, 2014).

Expected outcomes. End results that are measurable, desirable, and observable, and translate into observable behaviors.

Family. Family of origin or significant others as identified by the healthcare consumer.

Graduate-level prepared registered nurse. A registered nurse prepared at the master's or doctoral educational level who has advanced knowledge, skills, abilities, and judgment; functions in an advanced level as designated by elements of his or her position; and is not required to have additional regulatory oversight.

Health. An experience that is often expressed in terms of wellness and illness, and may occur in the presence or absence of disease or injury.

Healthcare consumer. The person, client, family, group, community, or population who is the focus of attention and to whom the registered nurse is providing services as sanctioned by the state regulatory bodies.

Healthcare providers. Individuals with special expertise who provide healthcare services or assistance to patients. They may include nurses, physicians, psychologists, social workers, nutritionist/dietitians, and various therapists.

Holistic care. The integration of body-mind-emotion-spirit-sexual-cultural-social-energetic-environmental principles and modalities to promote health, increase well-being, and actualize human potential.

Illness. The subjective experience of discomfort, disharmony, or imbalance. Not synonymous with disease.

Implementation. Activities such as teaching, monitoring, providing, counseling, delegating, and coordinating.

Information. Data that are interpreted, organized, or structured.

Interprofessional. Reliant on the overlapping knowledge, skills, and abilities of each professional team member. This can drive synergistic effects by which outcomes are enhanced and become more comprehensive than a simple aggregation of the individual efforts of the team members.

Interprofessional collaboration. Integrated enactment of knowledge, skills, and values and attitudes that define working together across the professions, with other healthcare workers, and with patients, along with families and communities, as appropriate to improve health outcomes (IECEP, 2011).

Nursing. The protection, promotion, and optimization of health and abilities, prevention of illness and injury, facilitation of healing, alleviation of suffering through the diagnosis and treatment of human response, and advocacy in the care of individuals, families, groups, communities, and populations.

Nursing practice. The collective professional activities of nurses characterized by the interrelations of human responses, theory application, nursing actions, and outcomes.

Nursing process. A critical thinking model used by nurses that is represented as the integration of the singular, concurrent actions of these six components: assessment, diagnosis, identification of outcomes, planning, implementation, and evaluation.

Patient. *See* Healthcare consumer

Peer review.   A collegial, systematic, and periodic process by which registered nurses are held accountable for practice and which fosters the refinement of one's knowledge, skills, and decision-making at all levels and in all areas of practice.

Plan.   A comprehensive outline of the components that need to be addressed to attain expected outcomes.

Quality.   The degree to which health services for patients, families, groups, communities, or populations increase the likelihood of desired outcomes and are consistent with current professional knowledge.

Registered nurse (RN).   An individual registered or licensed by a state, commonwealth, territory, government, or other regulatory body to practice as a registered nurse.

Scope of Nursing Practice.   The description of the *who, what, where, when, why,* and *how* of nursing practice that addresses the range of nursing practice activities common to all registered nurses. When considered in conjunction with the Standards of Professional Nursing Practice and the Code of Ethics for Nurses, comprehensively describes the competent level of nursing common to all registered nurses.

Standards.   Authoritative statements defined and promoted by the profession by which the quality of practice, service, or education can be evaluated.

Standards of Professional Nursing Practice.   Authoritative statements of the duties that all registered nurses, regardless of role, population, or specialty, are expected to perform competently.

Standards of Practice.   Standards that describe a competent level of nursing care as demonstrated by the nursing process. *See also* Nursing process.

Standards of Professional Performance.   Standards that describe a competent level of behavior in the professional role.

Wellness.   Integrated, congruent functioning aimed toward reaching one's highest potential (AHNA, 2013).

Worldview.   The way people look out at their universe and form a picture or value about their lives and the world around them (Leininger, 1995, p. 105). "Worldview includes one's relationship with nature, moral and ethical reasoning, social relationships, and magico-religious beliefs" (Purnell & Paulanka, 1998, p.3), among others.

References and Bibliography

All websites accurate as of June 29, 2015.

Accreditation Commission for Midwifery Education (ACME). (2010). *Criteria for programmatic accreditation*. Silver Spring: Author. Available from http://www.midwife.org/acmedocs/ ACME.Programmatic.Criteria.Final.June.2010.pdf

Agency for Healthcare Research and Quality. Retrieved from *TeamSTEPPS: Strategies and tools to enhance performance and patient safety* http://www.ahrq.gov/professionals/education/ curriculum-tools/teamstepps/

Agency for Healthcare Research and Quality. (2008). *TeamSTEPPS fundamentals course: module 2* [webpage]. Retrieved from http://www.ahrq.gov/professionals/education/curriculum-tools/teamstepps/instructor/fundamentals/module2/igteamstruct.html

American Academy of Nurse Practitioners (AANP). (2007). *Standards of practice for nurse practitioners*. Washington, DC: Author. http://www.aanp.org/NR/rdonlyres/FE00E81B-FA96-4779-972B-6162F04C309F/0/Standards_of_Practice112907.pdf

American Association of Colleges of Nursing (AACN). (2004). *AACN position statement on the practice doctorate in nursing*. October 2004. City of Publication: Author

American Association of Colleges of Nursing (AACN). (2005). *AACN standards for establishing and maintaining healthy work environments*. Mission Viejo, CA: AACN. Retrieved from http:// www.aacn.org/wd/hwe/docs/hwestandards.pdf

American Association of Colleges of Nursing. (AACN). (2008). *The essentials of baccalaureate education for professional nursing practice*. Washington, DC: Author

American Association of Colleges of Nursing (AACN). (2014). Nursing shortage. Retrieved from http://www.aacn.nche.edu/media-relations/fact-sheets/nursing-shortage.

American Association of Colleges of Nursing (AACN). (2015). Interdisciplinary education and practice. Retrieved from http://www.aacn.nche.edu/publications/position/ interdisciplinary-education-and-practice

American Association of Nurse Anesthetists (AANA). (2007). *Scope and standards for nurse anesthesia practice*. Park Ridge, IL: Author. http://www.aana.com/resources2/ professionalpractice/Documents/PPM%20Standards%20for%20Nurse%20Anesthesia%20 Practice.pdf

American College of Nurse-Midwives (ACNM). (2008). *Core competencies for basic midwifery practice*. Silver Spring: Author. Available at http://www.midwife.org/siteFiles/descriptive/ Core_Competencies_6_07_000.pdf

American College of Nurse-Midwives. (ACNM) (2009). *Standards for the practice of midwifery*. Silver Spring: Author. Available at http://www.midwife.org/siteFiles/descriptive/Standards_ for_Practice_of_Midwifery_12_09_001.pdf

American Journal of Nursing. (1911). Editorial comments. Room at the top. *12*(2), 85–90. (Available to subscribers only at http://journals.lww.com/ajnonline/toc/1911/11000)

American Nurses Association (2013c). *Competency Model.* ANA Leadership Institute, 2013. Retrieved from http://www.ana-leadershipinstitute.org/Doc-Vault/About-Us/ANA-Leadership-Institute-Competency-Model-pdf.pdf

American Nurses Association. (1980). *Nursing: A social policy statement.* Kansas City, MO: Author.

American Nurses Association. (1995). *Nursing's social policy statement.* Washington, DC: Author.

American Nurses Association (ANA). (2003). *Nursing's social policy statement* (2nd ed.). Silver Spring, MD: Nursesbooks.org

American Nurses Asssociation (ANA). (2006.) *Recognition of a nursing specialty, specialty nursing scope statement, and specialty nursing standards of practice.* Silver Spring, MD: Author.

American Nurses Association (ANA). (2007). *ANA principles of environmental health for nursing practice with implementation strategies.* Silver Spring, MD: Nursesbooks.org.

American Nurses Association (ANA). (2008). Elimination of manual patient handling to prevent work-related musculoskeletal disorders [webpage]. Retrieved from http://www.nursingworld.org/MainMenuCategories/Policy-Advocacy/Positions-and-Resolutions/ANAPositionStatements/Position-Statements-Alphabetically/Elimination-of-Manual-Patient-Handling-to-Prevent-Work-Related-Musculoskeletal-Disorders.html

American Nurses Association (ANA). (2010a). *Nursing: Scope and standards of practice* (2nd ed.). Silver Spring, MD: Nursesbooks.org.

American Nurses Association (ANA). (2010b). *Nursing's social policy statement: The essence of the profession.* Silver Spring, MD: Nursesbooks.org.

American Nurses Association (ANA). (2012a). *ANA's principles of nurse staffing.* Silver Spring, MD: Author.

American Nurses Association (ANA). (2012b). *Bullying and workplace violence.* Retrieved from http://nursingworld.org/MainMenuCategories/WorkplaceSafety/Healthy-Nurse/bullyingworkplaceviolence

American Nurses Association (ANA). (2012c). *Safe patient handling and mobility interprofessional standards.* Silver Spring, MD: Author.

American Nurses Association (ANA). (2013a). *Framework for measuring nurses' contributions to care coordination.* http://www.nursingworld.org/Framework-for-Measuring-Nurses-Contributions-to-Care-Coordination

American Nurses Association (ANA). (2013b). HealthyNurseTM [webpage]. Retrieved from http://www.nursingworld.org/MainMenuCategories/WorkplaceSafety/Healthy-Nurse

American Nurses Association (ANA). (2014a). Addressing nurse fatigue to promote safety and health: Joint responsibilities of registered nurses and employers to reduce risks [webpage]. Retrieved from http://www.nursingworld.org/MainMenuCategories/Policy-Advocacy/Positions-and-Resolutions/ANAPositionStatements/Position-Statements-Alphabetically/Addressing-Nurse-Fatigue-to-Promote-Safety-and-Health.html

American Nurses Association (ANA). (2014b). *Health care transformation: The Affordable Care Act and More.* Retrieved from http://nursingworld.org/MainMenuCategories/Policy-Advocacy/HealthSystemReform/AffordableCareAct.pdf

American Nurses Association (ANA). (2014c). Nurse staffing [webpage]. Retrieved from http://www.nursingworld.org/MainMenuCategories/ThePracticeofProfessionalNursing/NurseStaffing

American Nurses Association (ANA). (2014d). *Professional role competence (Position Statement).* Silver Spring, MD : Author.

American Nurses Asssociation (ANA). (2015). *Code of Ethics for Nurses with Interpretive Statements*. Silver Spring, MD: Nursesbooks.org

American Nurses Credentialing Center (ANCC). (2008). *A new model for ANCC's Magnet Recognition Program*. Silver Spring, MD: Author.

American Nurses Credentialing Center (ANCC). (2012). *Practice standards* [webpage]. Retrieved from http://www.nursecredentialing.org/Pathway/AboutPathway/PathwayPracticeStandards

American Nurses Credentialing Center (ANCC). (2014). Magnet Model. Retrieved from http://www.nursecredentialing.org/Magnet/ProgramOverview/New-Magnet-Model

Andrews, M. M. (forthcoming 2015). Theoretical foundations of transcultural nursing. In M. M. Andrews & J. S. Boyle (Eds.), *Transcultural concepts in nursing care*. Philadelphia: Wolters Kluwer/Lippincott, Williams, & Wilkins.

APRN Joint Dialogue Group. (2008.) *Consensus model for APRN regulation: Licensure, accreditation, certification and education.* Retrieved from http://www.nursingworld.org/ConsensusModelforAPRN

Benner, P. (1982). From novice to expert. *American Journal of Nursing, 82*(3), 402–407.

Board of Higher Education & Massachusetts Organization of Nurse Executives. (BHE/MONE). (2006). *Creativity and connections: Building the framework for the Future of Nursing Education. Report from the Invitational Working Session, March 23–24, 2006.* Burlington, MA: MONE. http://www.mass.edu/currentinit/documents/NursingCreativityAndConnections.pdf

Campinha-Bacote, J. (2011a). Coming to know cultural competence: An evolutionary process. *International Journal For Human Caring, 15*(3), 42–48.

Campinha-Bacote, J. (2011b). Delivering patient-centered care in the midst of a cultural conflict: The role of cultural competence. *The Online Journal of Issue in Nursing, 16*(2), Manuscript 5. Retrieved from http://gm6.nursingworld.org/MainMenuCategories/ANAMarketplace/ANAPeriodicals/OJIN/TableofContents/Vol-16-2011/No2-May-2011/Delivering-Patient-Centered-Care-in-the-Midst-of-a-Cultural-Conflict.aspx#Framework

Carper, B. (1978). Fundamental patterns of knowing in nursing. *Advances in Nursing Science, 1*(1), 13–23.

Centers for Disease Control and Prevention (CDC). (2014a). Health Expenditures. http://www.cdc.gov/nchs/fastats/health-expenditures.htm

Centers for Disease Control and Prevention (CDC). (2014b). Mortality in the United States, 2013. http://www.cdc.gov/nchs/data/databriefs/db178.htm

Central Intelligence Agency (CIA). (2014). The World Fact Book. https://www.cia.gov/library/publications/the-world-factbook/rankorder/2102rank.html

Cipriano, P. (2009) in IOM (Institute of Medicine). 2010. *A summary of the October 2009 forum on the future of nursing: Acute care.* Washington, DC: The National Academies Press.

Curtin, L. (2007). The perfect storm: Managed care, aging adults, and a nursing shortage. *Nursing Administration Quarterly, 31*(2), 105–114.

Department of Defense (2014). Military Health System (MHS) and Defense Health Agency (DHA). *TeamSTEPPS*. Retrieved from http://www.health.mil/Military-Health-Topics/Access-Cost-Quality-and-Safety/Quality-And-Safety-of-Healthcare/Patient-Safety/Patient-Safety-Products-And-Services/TeamSTEPPS

Douglas, M. K., Rosenkoetter, M., Pacquiao, D. F., Callister, L. C., Milstead, J., Nardi, D., & Purnell, L. (2014). Guidelines for implementing culturally competent nursing care. *Journal of Transcultural Nursing, 25*(2), 109–121. doi: 10.1177/1043659614520998.

Douglas, M. K., Pierce, J. U., Rosenkoetter, M., Pacquiao, D., Callister, L. C., Hattar-Pollara, M., Lauderdale, J., Milstead, D., Nardi, D., & Purnell, L. (2011). Standards of practice for culturally competent nursing care. *Journal of Transcultural Nursing, 22*(2), 109–121.

Earp, J. A., French, E. A., & Gilkey, M. B. (Eds.). (2008). *Patient advocacy for health care quality: Strategies for achieving patient-centered care.* Sudbury, MA: Jones and Bartlett Publishers.

Estabrooks C.A., D. S. Thompson, J.J. Lovely, & A. Hofmeyer. (2006). A guide to knowledge translation theory. *Journal of Continuing Education in the Health Professions* (1):25–36. Winter.

Eyre, E. (n.d.). *Forming, storming, norming, and performing: Understanding the stages of team formation.* Retrieved from http://www.mindtools.com/pages/article/newLDR_86.htm

Fineberg, H. V., Lavizzo-Mourney, R. (2013). The Future of Nursing: A Look Back at the Landmark IOM. Reporthttp://www.iom.edu/Global/Perspectives/2013/The-Future-of-Nursing.aspx

Finfgeld-Connett, D. (2006). Meta-synthesis of caring in nursing. *Journal of Clinical Nursing, 17,* 196–204.

Gallagher-Lepak, S., & Kubsch, S. (2009). Transpersonal caring: A nursing practice guideline. *Holistic Nursing Practice, 23,* 171–182.

Giger, J. N, & Davidhizar, R. E. (2008). *Transcultural nursing. Assessment and intervention* (5th ed.). St. Louis, Missouri: Mosby/Elsevier.

Hagerty, B. M. K., Lynch-Sauer, K., Patusky, K. L., & Bouwseman, M. (1993). An emerging theory of human relatedness. *Image, 25,* 291–296.

Hain, D., Fleck, L. M. (2014). Barriers to NP practice that impact healthcare redesign. *The Online Journal of Issues in Nursing* (OJIN). 19(2). http://www.nursingworld.org/MainMenuCategories/ANAMarketplace/ANAPeriodicals/OJIN/TableofContents/Vol-19-2014/No2-May-2014/Barriers-to-NP-Practice.html

Health Resources and Services Administration (HRSA). (2010). The registered nurse population: Findings from the 2008 national sample survey of registered nurses. Retrieved from http://bhpr.hrsa.gov/healthworkforce/rnsurveys/rnsurveyfinal.pdf

Huston, C. (2013). The impact of emerging technology on nursing care: Warp speed ahead. *Online Journal of Issues in Nursing,* 18(2), Manuscript 1. Retrieved from http://www.nursingworld.org/MainMenuCategories/ANAMarketplace/ANAPeriodicals/OJIN/TableofContents/Vol-18-2013/No2-May-2013/Impact-of-Emerging-Technology.html

Institute of Medicine (IOM). (1999). *To err is human: Building a safer health system.* Washington, DC: National Academies Press.

Institute of Medicine (IOM). (2001). *Crossing the quality chasm.* Washington, DC: National Academies Press.

Institute of Medicine (IOM). (2003). *Health professions education: A bridge to quality.* Washington, DC: National Academies Press.

Institute of Medicine (IOM). (2004). *Keeping patients safe: Transforming the work environment of nurses.* Washington, DC: National Academies Press.

Institute of Medicine (IOM). (2009). *Forum on the Future of Nursing: Acute care.* "Technology-Enabled Nursing" and "Reactions and Questions" in Chapter 4, Technology, pp.28–33. Washington, DC: National Academies Press. Available from http://www.nap.edu/catalog.php?record_id=12855

Institute of Medicine (IOM). (2010). *The future of nursing: Leading change, advancing health.* Washington, D.C.: National Academies Press.

Institute of Medicine (IOM). (2011). *The future of nursing: Focus on education.* Available at http://www.iom.edu/Reports/2010/The-Future-of-Nursing-Leading-Change-Advancing-Health/Report-Brief-Education.aspx.

Interprofessional Education Collaborative Expert Panel (IECEP). (2011). *Core competencies for interprofessional collaborative practice: Report of an expert panel.* Washington, D.C.:

Interprofessional Education Collaborative Expert Panel (IECEP). (2011). *Core competencies for interprofessional collaborative practice: Report of an expert panel.* Washington, D.C.: Interprofessional Education Collaborative. Also available online: http://www.aacn.nche.edu/education-resources/ipecreport.pdf

International Council of Nurses (ICN). (2012). *Closing the gap: From evidence to action.* ISBN: 978-92-95094-75-8. Retrieved from www.nursingworld.org/MainMenuCategories/ThePracticeofProfessionalNursing/Improving-Your-Practice/Research-Toolkit/ICN-Evidence-Based-Practice-Resource/Closing-the-Gap-from-Evidence-to-Action.pdf

Jeffreys, M. R. (2010). A model to guide cultural competence education. In M. R. Jeffreys (Ed.), *Teaching cultural competence in nursing and health care: Inquiry, action, and innovation* (2nd ed., pp. 45–59). New York: Springer.

The Joint Commission (2012). *Hot topics in health care: Transitions of care: The need for a more effective approach to continuing patient care.* Author: Oakbrook Terrace, IL. Retrieved from http://www.jointcommission.org/assets/1/18/Hot_Topics_Transitions_of_Care.pdf

Joynt, J., & Kimball, B. (2008). *Blowing open the bottleneck: Designing new approaches to increase nurse education capacity.* Princeton, NJ: Robert Wood Johnson Foundation.

Kane, R. L., Shamilyan, T., Mueller, C., Duval, S., & Wilt, T. J. (2007). *Nurse staffing and quality of patient care.* Rockville, MD: Agency for Healthcare Research and Quality.

Lamb, G. (2014). *Care coordination: The game changer: How nursing is revolutionizing quality care.* Silver Spring, MD: Nursesbooks.org.

Leininger, M. (1988). Leininger's Theory of Nursing: Cultural care diversity and universality. *Nursing Science Quarterly, 1*(4), 152–160.

Leininger, M. (1995). *Transcultural nursing. Concepts, theories, research & practices* (2nd ed.). New York: McGraw-Hill, Inc.

Leininger, M. M., & McFarland, M. R. (2002). *Transcultural nursing: Concepts, theories, research and practice.* n.p.: McGraw-Hill Education.

McFarland, M. R., & Wehbe-Alamah, H. B. (2015). The theory of culture care diversity and universality. In M. R. McFarland and H. B. Wehbe-Alamah (Eds.), *Leininger's culture care diversity and universality: A worldwide nursing theory* (3rd ed., p. 25). Burlington, MA: Jones and Bartlett Learning.

McMenamin, P. (2015). ANA: voice of 3.4 million nurses—and growing. One Strong Voice. (American Nurses Association's health policy blog). Retrieved from http://www.ananursespace.org/blogs/peter-mcmenamin/2015/06/29/ana

Melnyk, B. M., & Fineout-Overholt, E. (2011). *Evidence-based practice in nursing & healthcare: A guide to best practice (2nd ed.).* New York: Lippincott, Williams & Wilkins.

Melnyk B. M., L. Gallagher-Ford, L. E. Long , & E. Fineout-Overholt (2014). The establishment of evidence-based practice competencies for practicing registered nurses and advanced practice nurses in real-world clinical settings: proficiencies to improve healthcare quality, reliability, patient outcomes, and costs. *Worldviews Evidence-Based Nursing* 11(1):5–15 (February). doi: 10.1111/wvn.12021. (Epub 2014 Jan 21.)

Mitchell, P., Wynia, M., Golden, R., McNellis, B., Okun, S., Webb, C., Rohrbach, V., & Von Kohorn, I. (2012 October). Institute of Medicine: *Core principles and values of effective team-based health care.* Discussion paper, IOM Roundtable on Value & Science-Driven Health Care. June 2012. Washington, DC: Institute of Medicine.

Moffitt, Phillip (2004), in M. Koloroutis (ed.) *Relationship-based care: A model for transforming practice.* Minneapolis: Creative Health Care Management.

Moorhead, Sue, Marion Johnson, Meridean L. Maas, & Elizabeth Swanson (2012). *Nursing Outcomes Classification (NOC): Measurement of health outcomes* 5th ed. Maryland Heights; MO: Mosby.

National Association of Clinical Nurse Specialists (NACNS). (2009). *Core practice doctorate clinical nurse specialist (CNS) competencies.* Philadelphia: Author. Retrieved from http://www.nacns.org/docs/CorePracticeDoctorate.pdf

National Association of Clinical Nurse Specialists (NACNS). (2010). *Organizing framework and CNS core competencies.* Philadelphia: Author. Retrieved from http://www.nacns.org/docs/CNSCoreCompetenciesBroch.pdf

National Institute for Occupational Safety and Health (NIOSH). (2013a). Occupational violence training and education [web course]. Available at http://www.cdc.gov/niosh/topics/violence/training_nurses.html

National Institute for Occupational Safety and Health (NIOSH). (2013b). Traumatic injury: NIOSH research projects [webpage]. Retrieved from http://www.cdc.gov/niosh/programs/ti/projects.html

National Organization of Nurse Practitioner Faculties (NONPF). (2006). *Domains and core competencies of nurse practitioner practice.* Washington, DC: Author. http://c.ymcdn.com/sites/www.nonpf.org/resource/resmgr/competencies/domainsandcorecomps2006.pdf

Newhouse, R. P. (2010). Do we know how much the evidence-based intervention cost? *Journal of Nursing Administration, 40*(7/8), 296–299.

Nightingale, F. (1859). *Notes on nursing.* New York: Dover Publications.

OECD (2013), *Health at a glance 2013: OECD Indicators.* OECD Publishing. http://dx.doi.org/10.1787/health_glance-2013-en

Organization for Economic Cooperation and Development (OECD). (2014). Health Status: Life expectancy at birth [webpage]. Retrieved from http://data.oecd.org/healthstat/life-expectancy.htm

Paley, J. (2002). Caring as slave morality: Nietzchean themes in nursing ethics. *Journal of Advanced Nursing, 40*(1), 25–35.

Pentland, A. (2012). The new science of building great teams. *Harvard Business Review, 90*(4), 60–69.

Purnell, L. (2013). The Purnell model for cultural competence. In L. Purnell (Ed.), *Transcultural health care: A culturally competent approach* (pp. 15–44). Philadelphia: F. A. Davis Co.

Purnell, L. D., & Paulanka, B. J. (1998). *Transcultural health care: A culturally competent approach.* Philadelphia: F. A. Davis, Co.

Quinn, J. (2013). Transpersonal human caring and healing. In B. Dossey and L. Keegan (Eds.), *Holistic nursing: A handbook for practice, 6th ed.* (pp. 107–116). Sudbury, MA: Jones & Bartlett.

Robert Wood Johnson Foundation (RWJF). (2014). Campaign helps advance institute of medicine's call for more nurse leaders. *Sharing Nursing's Knowledge*, October 2014. Retrieved from http://www.rwjf.org/en/library/articles-and-news/2014/10/campaign-helps-advance-institute-of-medicine-s-call-for-more-nur.html

Robert Wood Johnson Foundation (RWJF) & Institute of Medicine (IOM). (2009). *Robert Wood Johnson Foundation, Institute of Medicine launch unprecedented initiative on the future of nursing in America.* Princeton, NJ: RWJF. Retrieved from http://www.rwjf.org/pr/product.jsp?id=45714

Samueli Institute. (2010). *Optimal healing environments* [webpage]. Retrieved from https://www.samueliinstitute.org/research-areas/optimal-healing-environments

Spector, Rachel E. (2013). *Cultural diversity in health and illness* (8th ed.). Upper Saddle River, NJ: Prentice Hall, Inc.

Stewart, I. M. (1948). *The education of nurses: Historical foundations and modern trends.* New York: Macmillan Company.

Swanson, K. (1993). Empirical development of a middle-range theory of caring. *Nursing Research, 40*(3), 161–166.

Styles, M. M., Schumann, M. J., Bickford, C. J., & White, K. M. (2008). *Specialization and credentialing in nursing revisited: Understanding the issues, advancing the profession.* Silver Spring, MD: Nursesbooks.org.

Tri-Regulator Collaborative (2014). The Tri-Regulator Collaborative Position Statement on interprofessional, team-based patient care. Retrieved from https://www.ncsbn.org/Team-Based_Care.pdf

Trust for America's Health. (2009). *Making the case: prevention and health reform.* Washington, DC: Author. http://healthyamericans.org/assets/files/5.20.09PreventionandReformTPs.pdf

U.S. Congress. House of Representatives. (June 25, 2013). *H.R.2480 - Nurse and Health Care Worker Protection Act of 2013.* Washington, DC: U.S. Government Printing Office. Retrieved from https://www.congress.gov/bill/113th-congress/house-bill/2480.

U.S. Bureau of Labor Statistics (BLS). (2010.) *Occupational outlook handbook, 2010–11 Edition. Registered nurses.* Washington, DC: Author. Retrieved from http://www.bls.gov/ooh/healthcare/registered-nurses.htm

U.S. Bureau of Labor Statistics (BLS). (2013). Table 8. Occupations with the largest projected number of job openings due to growth and replacement needs, 2012 and projected 2022 [webpage]. Retrieved from http://www.bls.gov/news.release/ecopro.t08.htm

U.S. Bureau of Labor Statistics (BLS). (2014). "29-1141 Registered Nurses." Retrieved from http://www.bls.gov/oes/current/oes291141.htm

Watson, J. (2008). *Assessing and measuring caring in nursing and health sciences* (2nd ed.). New York: Springer Publishing Co.

Watson, J. (2012). *Human caring science: A theory of nursing* (2nd ed.). Sudbury, MA: Jones and Bartlett Learning.

Watts, S., Gee, J., O'Day, M., Schaub, K., Lawrence, R., & Kirsch, S. (2009). "Nurse practitioner-led multidisciplinary teams to improve chronic illness care: The unique strengths of nurse practitioners applied to shared medical appointments/group visits." *Journal of the Association of American Academic Nurse Practitioners* 21(3): 167–72. doi: 10.1111/j.1745-7599.2008.00379.x.

Weston, M., & Roberts, D. W. (2013). The influence of quality improvement efforts on patient outcomes and nursing work: A perspective from chief nursing officers at three large health systems. *The Online Journal of Issues in Nursing, 18*(3), Manuscript 2. Retrieved from http://www.nursingworld.org/MainMenuCategories/ANAMarketplace/ANAPeriodicals/OJIN/TableofContents/Vol-18-2013/No3-Sept-2013/Quality-Improvement-on-Patient-Outcomes.html

Appendix A
Nursing: Scope and Standards of Practice, 2nd Edition (2010)

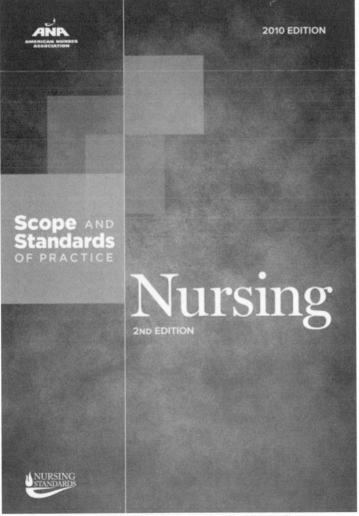

The content of the selected pages reproduced in this appendix are
not current and is of historical significance only.

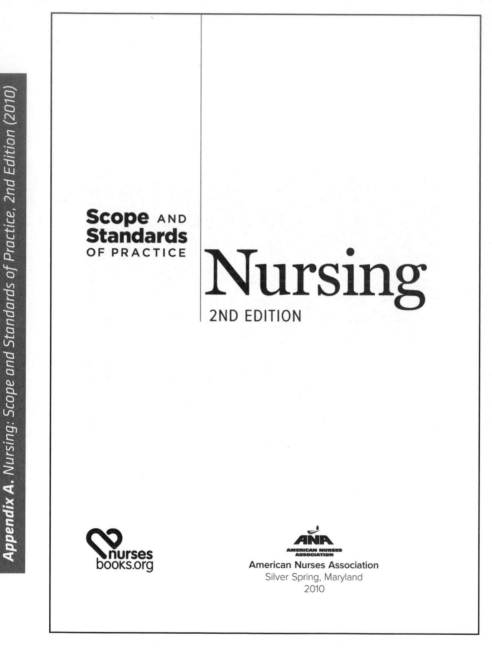

Scope AND
Standards
OF PRACTICE

Nursing

2ND EDITION

nurses
books.org

American Nurses Association
Silver Spring, Maryland
2010

The content in this appendix is not current and is of historical significance only.

Contents

iii

Appendix A. Nursing: Scope and Standards of Practice, 2nd Edition (2010)

Appendix A. Nursing: Scope and Standards of Practice, 2nd Edition (2010)

The content in this appendix is not current and is of historical significance only.

CONTENTS

Appendix A. Nursing: Scope and Standards of Practice, 2nd Edition (2010)

Contributors

Nursing: Scope and Standards of Practice, Second Edition is the product of significant thought work by many registered nurses and a four-step review process involving those listed below. The document originated from the decisions garnered during a significant number of telephone conference calls and electronic mail communications of the diverse workgroup members, then followed by an extensive public comment period. The review process included two evaluations by the Committee on Nursing Practice Standards and Guidelines of ANA's Congress on Nursing Practice and Economics, review and approval by the entire Congress on Nursing Practice and Economics, and finally, review and approval by the American Nurses Association Board of Directors in May 2010. The list of endorsing organizations that completes this section reflects the broad acceptance of this resource within the profession.

Nursing Scope and Standards Workgroup, 2009–2010

Ann O'Sullivan, MSN, RN, NE-BC, CNE – Chair
  Julia Rose Barcott, RN
  Nancy Bonalumi, MS, RN, CEN, FAEN
  Susan B. Collins, FNP-BC, AHN-BC
  Louise Darling, BSN, RNC, IBCLC
  Gwen A. Davis, MN, RN, CDE
  Melanie Duffy, MSN, RN, CCRN, CCNS
  Diane Earl, RN
  Janice Cooke Feigenbaum, PhD, RN
  Jacqueline Fournier, APRN, BC
  Michael J. Kremer, PhD, CRNA, FAAN

vii

Kathleen A.V. Lavery, MS, CNM
Beth Martin, MSN, RN, CCNS, ACNP-BC, ACHP
Deborah Maust Martin, MSN, RN, MBA, NE-BC, FACHE
Mary-Anne Ponti, MSN, MBA, RN, CNAA-BC
Harry F. Smith, CDR, NC, USN
Juan Carlos Soto, EdD, MSN, RN
Cindy Diamond Zolnierek, MSN, RN

(For more about the workgroup, go to this book's record at
www.Nursesbooks.org.)

ANA Staff, 2009–2010

Carol J. Bickford, PhD, RN-BC	Content editor
Katherine C. Brewer, MSN, RN	Content editor
Maureen E. Cones, Esq.	Legal counsel
Yvonne Humes, MSA	Project coordinator
Eric Wurzbacher	Project editor

Committee on Nursing Practice Standards and Guidelines. 2009–2010

Tresha L. Lucas, MSN, RN, CNAA-BC – Chair
Rosemary Pais Brown, MSN, RN
Julia A. Dangel, MSN, RN
Judith Harris, EdD, ARNP
Richard Henker, PhD, RN, CRNA
Wanda Lewis, DHA, RN, CCRN
Sandi McDermott, RN, MSN, NEA-BC
Margaret Nelson, MS, RN
Elizabeth Libby Thomas, Med, RN, NCSN, FNASN

Congress on Nursing Practice and Economics, 2008–2010

CHAIR
Kathleen M. White, PhD, RN, CNAA-BC

VICE-CHAIR
Ann M. O'Sullivan, RN, MSN, NE-BC, CNE

Appendix A. Nursing: Scope and Standards of Practice, 2nd Edition (2010)

Overview of the Content

Foundational Documents of Professional Nursing

Registered nurses practicing in the United States have three professional resources that inform their thinking and decision-making and guide their practice. First, *Code of Ethics for Nurses with Interpretive Statements* (ANA, 2001) lists the nine succinct provisions that establish the ethical framework for registered nurses across all roles, levels, and settings. Second, *Nursing's Social Policy Statement: The Essence of the Profession* (ANA, 2010) conceptualizes nursing practice, describes the social context of nursing, and provides the definition of nursing.

Nursing: Scope and Standards of Practice, Second Edition, outlines the expectations of the professional role of the registered nurse. It states the scope of practice and presents the standards of professional nursing practice and their accompanying competencies.

Additional Content

For a better appreciation of the history and context related to *Nursing: Scope and Standards of Practice, Second Edition*, readers will find the additional content of the four appendixes useful:

- Appendix A. ANA's Principles of Environmental Health for Nursing Practice

xvii

- Appendix B. Professional Role Competence: ANA Position Statement
- Appendix C. The Development of Foundational Nursing Documents and Professional Nursing
- Appendix D. Nursing: Scope and Standards of Practice (2004)

Audience for This Publication

Registered nurses in every role and setting constitute the primary audience of this professional resource. Legislators, regulators, legal counsel, and the judiciary system will also want to reference it. Agencies, organizations, nurse administrators, and interprofessional colleagues will find this an invaluable reference. In addition, the people, families, communities, and populations using healthcare and nursing services can use this document to better understand what constitutes nursing and who its members are: registered nurses and advanced practice registered nurses

Appendix A. Nursing: Scope and Standards of Practice, 2nd Edition (2010)

Scope of Nursing Practice

Definition of Nursing

Nursing's Social Policy Statement: The Essence of the Profession (ANA, 2010, p. 3) builds on previous work and provides the following contemporary definition of nursing:

> *Nursing is the protection, promotion, and optimization of health and abilities, prevention of illness and injury, alleviation of suffering through the diagnosis and treatment of human response, and advocacy in the care of individuals, families, communities, and populations.*

This definition serves as the foundation for the following expanded description of the Scope of Nursing Practice and the Standards of Professional Nursing Practice.

Professional Nursing's Scope and Standards of Practice

A professional nursing organization has a responsibility to its members and to the public it serves to develop the scope and standards of its profession's practice. As the professional organization for all registered nurses, the American Nurses Association (ANA) has assumed the responsibility for developing the scope and standards that apply to the practice of all professional nurses and serve as a template for nursing specialty practice. Standards do, however, belong

1

to the profession and, thus, require broad input into their development and revision. *Nursing: Scope and Standards of Practice, Second Edition,* describes a competent level of nursing practice and professional performance common to all registered nurses.

Description of the Scope of Nursing Practice

The scope of practice statement describes the "who," "what," "where," "when," "why," and "how" of nursing practice. Each of these questions must be answered to provide a complete picture of the dynamic and complex practice of nursing and its evolving boundaries and membership. The profession of nursing has one scope of practice that encompasses the full range of nursing practice, pertinent to general and specialty practice. The depth and breadth in which individual registered nurses engage in the total scope of nursing practice are dependent on their education, experience, role, and the population served.

Development and Function of Nursing Standards

The Standards of Professional Nursing Practice are authoritative statements of the duties that all registered nurses, regardless of role, population, or specialty, are expected to perform competently. The standards published herein may serve as evidence of the standard of care, with the understanding that application of the standards depends on context. The standards are subject to change with the dynamics of the nursing profession, as new patterns of professional practice are developed and accepted by the nursing profession and the public. In addition, specific conditions and clinical circumstances may also affect the application of the standards at a given time, e.g., during a natural disaster. The standards are subject to formal, periodic review and revision.

The Function of Competencies in Standards

The competencies that accompany each standard may be evidence of compliance with the corresponding standard. The list of competencies is not exhaustive. Whether a particular standard or competency applies depends upon the circumstances. For example, a nurse providing treatment to an unconscious, critical patient who presented to the hospital by ambulance without family has a duty to collect comprehensive data pertinent to the patient's health (Standard 1. Assessment). However, under the attendant circumstances, that nurse may not be expected to assess family dynamics and impact on the patient's health and wellness (Assessment Competency). In the same circumstance, Standard 5B. Health Teaching and Health Promotion may not apply at all.

2   *Nursing: Scope and Standards of Practice, 2nd Edition*

The Nursing Process

The *nursing process* is often conceptualized as the integration of singular actions of assessment, diagnosis, and identification of outcomes, planning, implementation, and finally, evaluation. The nursing process in practice is not linear as often conceptualized, with a feedback loop from evaluation to assessment. Rather, it relies heavily on the bi-directional feedback loops from each component, as illustrated in Figure 1.

The Standards of Practice coincide with the steps of the nursing process to represent the directive nature of the standards as the professional nurse completes each component of the nursing process. Similarly, the Standards of Professional Performance relate to how the professional nurse adheres to the Standards of Practice, completes the nursing process, and addresses other nursing practice issues and concerns (ANA, 2010). Five tenets characterize contemporary nursing practice (see next two pages).

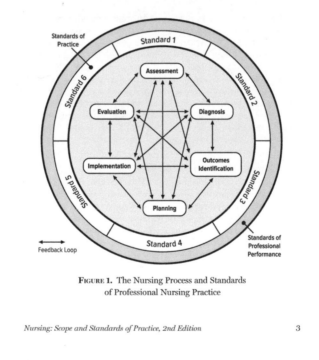

FIGURE 1. The Nursing Process and Standards of Professional Nursing Practice

Nursing: Scope and Standards of Practice, 2nd Edition 3

The content in this appendix is not current and is of historical significance only.

Appendix A. Nursing: Scope and Standards of Practice, 2nd Edition (2010)

Tenets Characteristic of Nursing Practice.

1. Nursing practice is individualized.

Nursing practice respects diversity and is individualized to meet the unique needs of the healthcare consumer or situation. *Healthcare consumer* is defined to be the patient, person, client, family, group, community, or population who is the focus of attention and to whom the registered nurse is providing services as sanctioned by the state regulatory bodies.

2. Nurses coordinate care by establishing partnerships.

The registered nurse establishes partnerships with persons, families, support systems, and other providers, utilizing in-person and electronic communications, to reach a shared goal of delivering health care. Health care is defined as the attempt "to address the health needs of the patient and the public" (ANA, 2001, p. 10). Collaborative interprofessional team planning is based on recognition of each discipline's value and contributions, mutual trust, respect, open discussion, and shared decision-making.

3. Caring is central to the practice of the registered nurse.

Professional nursing promotes healing and health in a way that builds a relationship between nurse and patient (Watson, 1999, 2008). "Caring is a conscious judgment that manifests itself in concrete acts, interpersonally, verbally, and nonverbally" (Gallagher-Lepak & Kubsch, 2009, p. 171). While caring for individuals, families, and populations is the key focus of nursing, the nurse additionally promotes self-care as well as care of the environment and society (Hagerty, Lynch-Sauer, Patusky, & Bouwseman, 1993).

4. Registered nurses use the nursing process to plan and provide individualized care to their healthcare consumers.

Nurses use theoretical and evidence-based knowledge of human experiences and responses to collaborate with healthcare consumers to assess, diagnose, identify outcomes, plan, implement, and evaluate care. Nursing interventions are intended to produce beneficial effects, contribute to quality outcomes, and above all, do no harm. Nurses evaluate the effectiveness of their care in relation to identified outcomes and use evidence-based practice to improve care (ANA,

2010). Critical thinking underlies each step of the nursing process, problem-solving, and decision-making. The nursing process is cyclical and dynamic, interpersonal and collaborative, and universally applicable.

5. A strong link exists between the professional work environment and the registered nurse's ability to provide quality health care and achieve optimal outcomes.

Professional nurses have an ethical obligation to maintain and improve health-care practice environments conducive to the provision of quality health care (ANA, 2001). Extensive studies have demonstrated the relationship between effective nursing practice and the presence of a healthy work environment. Mounting evidence demonstrates that negative, demoralizing, and unsafe conditions in the workplace (unhealthy work environments) contribute to medical errors, ineffective delivery of care, and conflict and stress among health professionals.

Healthy Work Environments for Nursing Practice

ANA supports the following models of healthy work environment design:

AMERICAN ASSOCIATION OF CRITICAL-CARE NURSES

The American Association of Critical-Care Nurses has identified six standards for establishing and maintaining healthy work environments (AACN, 2005):

- *Skilled Communication*
  Nurses must be as proficient in communication skills as they are in clinical skills.

- *True Collaboration*
  Nurses must be relentless in pursuing and fostering a sense of team and partnership across all disciplines.

- *Effective Decision-making*
  Nurses are seen as valued and committed partners in making policy, directing and evaluating clinical care, and leading organizational operations.

Nursing: Scope and Standards of Practice, 2nd Edition　　　　5

- *Appropriate Staffing*
  Staffing must ensure the effective match between healthcare consumer needs and nurse competencies.

- *Meaningful Recognition*
  Nurses must be recognized and must recognize others for the value each brings to the work of the organization.

- *Authentic Leadership*
  Nurse leaders must fully embrace the imperative of a healthy work environment, authentically live it, and engage others in achieving it.

MAGNET RECOGNITION PROGRAM

The Magnet Recognition Program® addresses the professional work environment, requiring that Magnet®-designated facilities adhere to the following model components (ANCC, 2008):

- *Transformational Leadership*
  The transformational leader leads people where they need to be in order to meet the demands of the future.

- *Structural Empowerment*
  Structures and processes developed by influential leadership provide an innovative practice environment in which strong professional practice flourishes and the mission, vision, and values come to life to achieve the outcomes believed to be important for the organization.

- *Exemplary Professional Practice*
  This demonstrates what professional nursing practice can achieve.

- *New Knowledge, Innovation, and Improvements*
  Organizations have an ethical and professional responsibility to contribute to healthcare delivery, the organization, and the profession.

- *Empirical Quality Results*
  Organizations are in a unique position to become pioneers of the future and to demonstrate solutions to numerous problems inherent in today's healthcare systems. Beyond the "What" and "How," organizations must ask themselves what difference these efforts have made

INSTITUTE OF MEDICINE

The Institute of Medicine has also reported that safety and quality problems occur when dedicated health professionals work in systems that neither support them nor prepare them to achieve optimal patient care outcomes (IOM, 2004). Such rapid changes as reimbursement modification and cost containment efforts, new healthcare technologies, and changes in the healthcare workforce have influenced the work and work environment of nurses. Accordingly, concentration on key aspects of the work environment—people, physical surroundings, and tools—can enhance healthcare working conditions and improve patient safety. These include:

- Transformational leadership and evidence-based management

- Maximizing workforce capability

- Creating and sustaining a culture of safety and research

- Work space design and redesign to prevent and mitigate errors

- Effective use of telecommunications and biomedical device interoperability

Appendix A. Nursing: Scope and Standards of Practice, 2nd Edition (2010)

The content in this appendix is not current and is of historical significance only.

Model of Professional Nursing Practice Regulation

In 2006 the Model of Professional Nursing Practice Regulation (see Figure 2) emerged from ANA work and informed the discussions of specialty nursing and advanced practice registered nurse practice.

The lowest level in the model represents the responsibility of the professional and specialty nursing organizations to their members and the public to define the scope and standards of practice for nursing.

The next level up the pyramid represents the regulation provided by the nurse practice acts and the rules and regulations in the pertinent licensing juris-

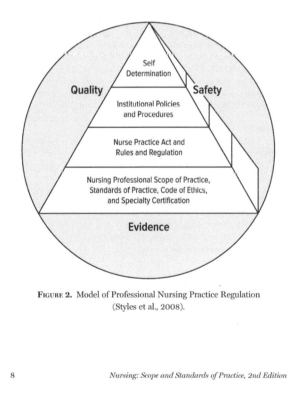

FIGURE 2. Model of Professional Nursing Practice Regulation
(Styles et al., 2008).

8   *Nursing: Scope and Standards of Practice, 2nd Edition*

Appendix A. Nursing: Scope and Standards of Practice, 2nd Edition (2010)

dictions. Institutional policies and procedures provide further considerations in the regulation of nursing practice for the registered nurse and advanced practice registered nurse.

Note that the highest level is that of self determination by the nurse after consideration of all the other levels of input about professional nursing practice regulation. The outcome is safe, quality, and evidence-based practice.

Standards of Professional Nursing Practice

The Standards of Professional Nursing Practice content consists of the Standards of Practice and the Standards of Professional Performance.

Standards of Practice

The Standards of Practice describe a competent level of nursing care as demonstrated by the critical thinking model known as the nursing process. The nursing process includes the components of assessment, diagnosis, outcomes identification, planning, implementation, and evaluation. Accordingly, the nursing process encompasses significant actions taken by registered nurses and forms the foundation of the nurse's decision-making.

STANDARD 1. ASSESSMENT
The registered nurse collects comprehensive data pertinent to the healthcare consumer's health and/or the situation.

STANDARD 2. DIAGNOSIS
The registered nurse analyzes the assessment data to determine the diagnoses or the issues.

STANDARD 3. OUTCOMES IDENTIFICATION
The registered nurse identifies expected outcomes for a plan individualized to the healthcare consumer or the situation.

STANDARD 4. PLANNING
The registered nurse develops a plan that prescribes strategies and alternatives to attain expected outcomes.

Nursing: Scope and Standards of Practice, 2nd Edition   9

The content in this appendix is not current and is of historical significance only.

STANDARD 5. IMPLEMENTATION
The registered nurse implements the identified plan.

STANDARD 5A. COORDINATION OF CARE
The registered nurse coordinates care delivery.

STANDARD 5B. HEALTH TEACHING AND HEALTH PROMOTION
The registered nurse employs strategies to promote health and a safe environment.

STANDARD 5C. CONSULTATION
The graduate-level prepared specialty nurse or advanced practice registered nurse provides consultation to influence the identified plan, enhance the abilities of others, and effect change.

STANDARD 5D. PRESCRIPTIVE AUTHORITY AND TREATMENT
The advanced practice registered nurse uses prescriptive authority, procedures, referrals, treatments, and therapies in accordance with state and federal laws and regulations.

STANDARD 6. EVALUATION
The registered nurse evaluates progress toward attainment of outcomes.

Standards of Professional Performance

The Standards of Professional Performance describe a competent level of behavior in the professional role, including activities related to ethics, education, evidence-based practice and research, quality of practice, communication, leadership, collaboration, professional practice evaluation, resource utilization, and environmental health. All registered nurses are expected to engage in professional role activities, including leadership, appropriate to their education and position. Registered nurses are accountable for their professional actions to themselves, their healthcare consumers, their peers, and ultimately to society.

Appendix A. *Nursing: Scope and Standards of Practice, 2nd Edition (2010)*

STANDARD 7. ETHICS
The registered nurse practices ethically.

STANDARD 8. EDUCATION
The registered nurse attains knowledge and competence that reflects current nursing practice.

STANDARD 9. EVIDENCE-BASED PRACTICE AND RESEARCH
The registered nurse integrates evidence and research findings into practice.

STANDARD 10. QUALITY OF PRACTICE
The registered nurse contributes to quality nursing practice.

STANDARD 11. COMMUNICATION
The registered nurse communicates effectively in all areas of practice.

STANDARD 12. LEADERSHIP
The registered nurse demonstrates leadership in the professional practice setting and the profession.

STANDARD 13. COLLABORATION
The registered nurse collaborates with healthcare consumer, family, and others in the conduct of nursing practice.

STANDARD 14. PROFESSIONAL PRACTICE EVALUATION
The registered nurse evaluates her or his own nursing practice in relation to professional practice standards and guidelines, relevant statutes, rules, and regulations.

STANDARD 15. RESOURCE UTILIZATION
The registered nurse utilizes appropriate resources to plan and provide nursing services that are safe, effective, and financially responsible.

STANDARD 16. ENVIRONMENTAL HEALTH
The registered nurse practices in an environmentally safe and healthy manner.

Nursing: Scope and Standards of Practice, 2nd Edition   11

Professional Competence in Nursing Practice

The public has a right to expect registered nurses to demonstrate professional competence throughout their careers. The registered nurse is individually responsible and accountable for maintaining professional competence. It is the nursing profession's responsibility to shape and guide any process for assuring nurse competence. Regulatory agencies define minimal standards of competency to protect the public. The employer is responsible and accountable to provide a practice environment conducive to competent practice. Assurance of competence is the shared responsibility of the profession, individual nurses, professional organizations, credentialing and certification entities, regulatory agencies, employers, and other key stakeholders (ANA, 2008).

ANA believes that in the practice of nursing competence can be defined, measured, and evaluated. No single evaluation method or tool can guarantee competence. Competence is situational and dynamic; it is both an outcome and an ongoing process. Context determines what competencies are necessary.

Definitions and Concepts Related to Competence

A number of terms are central to the discussion of competence:

- An individual who demonstrates "competence" is performing at an expected level.

- A *competency* is an expected level of performance that integrates knowledge, skills, abilities, and judgment.

- The integration of knowledge, skills, abilities, and judgment occurs in formal, informal, and reflective learning experiences.

- Knowledge encompasses thinking, understanding of science and humanities, professional standards of practice, and insights gained from context, practical experiences, personal capabilities, and leadership performance.

- Skills include psychomotor, communication, interpersonal, and diagnostic skills.

- Ability is the capacity to act effectively. It requires listening, integrity, knowledge of one's strengths and weaknesses, positive self-regard, emotional intelligence, and openness to feedback.

Appendix A. Nursing: Scope and Standards of Practice, 2nd Edition (2010)

- Judgment includes critical thinking, problem solving, ethical reasoning, and decision-making.

- *Formal learning* most often occurs in structured, academic, and professional development practice environments, while informal learning can be described as experiential insights gained in work, community, home, and other settings.

- *Reflective learning* represents the recurrent thoughtful personal self-assessment, analysis, and synthesis of strengths and opportunities for improvement. Such insights should lead to the creation of a specific plan for professional development and may become part of one's professional portfolio (ANA, 2008).

Competence and Competency in Nursing Practice

Competent registered nurses can be influenced by the nature of the situation, which includes consideration of the setting, resources, and the person. Situations can either enhance or detract from the nurse's ability to perform. The registered nurse influences factors that facilitate and enhance competent practice. Similarly, the nurse seeks to deal with barriers that constrain competent practice. The expected level of performance reflects variability depending upon context and the selected competence framework or model.

The ability to perform at the expected level requires a process of lifelong learning. Registered nurses must continually reassess their competencies and identify needs for additional knowledge, skills, personal growth, and integrative learning experiences.

Evaluating Competence

"Competence in nursing practice must be evaluated by the individual nurse (self-assessment), nurse peers, and nurses in the roles of supervisor, coach, mentor, or preceptor. In addition, other aspects of nursing performance may be evaluated by professional colleagues and patients.

Competence can be evaluated by using tools that capture objective and subjective data about the individual's knowledge base and actual performance and are appropriate for the specific situation and the desired outcome of the competence evaluation . . . However, no single evaluation tool or method can guarantee competence" (ANA, 2008, p. 6).

Appendix A. Nursing: Scope and Standards of Practice, 2nd Edition (2010)

The content in this appendix is not current and is of historical significance only.

Professional Registered Nurses Today

Statistical Snapshot

In 2008, there were an estimated 3 million registered nurses (RNs) in the United States, of which 2.6 million are currently employed. The majority of registered nurses initially entered nursing with an associate degree; however, the percentage of nurses entering practice with a bachelor's degree or higher has increased steadily. Most registered nurses work in hospitals (62%) and identify themselves as "staff nurses" (66%).

In addition to hospitals, nurses report working in ambulatory care (10%), public/community health (7.8%), home health (6.4%), nursing home/extended care (5.3%), academic education (3.8%), and other areas, including insurance, benefits, and utilization review (3.9%). Public/community health includes school and occupational health settings, and ambulatory care includes medical and physician practices, health centers and clinics, and other types of non-hospital clinic settings.

About 9% of nurses identify themselves as one of the four recognized advanced practice registered nurse roles, and other identified roles include management, patient coordinator, instructor, patient educator, and researcher. (U.S. Dept. of Labor, 2010; U.S. DHHS, 2010)

Licensure and Education of Registered Nurses

The registered nurse is licensed and authorized by a state, commonwealth, or territory to practice nursing. Professional licensure of the healthcare professions is established by each jurisdiction to protect the public safety and authorize the practice of the profession. Because of this, the requirements for RN licensure and advanced practice nursing vary widely.

The registered nurse is educationally prepared for competent practice at the beginning level upon graduation from an accredited school of nursing and qualified by national examination for RN licensure. ANA has consistently affirmed the baccalaureate degree in nursing as the preferred educational preparation for entry into nursing practice.

The registered nurse is educated in the art and science of nursing, with the goal of helping individuals and groups attain, maintain, and restore health whenever possible. Experienced nurses may become proficient in one or more practice areas or roles. These nurses may concentrate on healthcare consumer care in clinical nursing practice specialties. Others influence nursing and support the direct care rendered to healthcare consumers by those professional

14   *Nursing: Scope and Standards of Practice, 2nd Edition*

Appendix A. Nursing: Scope and Standards of Practice, 2nd Edition (2010)

nurses in clinical practice. Credentialing is one form of acknowledging such specialized knowledge and experience. Credentialing organizations may mandate specific nursing educational requirements, as well as timely demonstrations of knowledge and experience in specialty practice.

Registered nurses may pursue advanced academic studies to prepare for specialization in practice. Educational requirements vary by specialty and educational program. New models for educational preparation are evolving in response to the changing healthcare, education, and regulatory practice environments.

Roots of Professional Nursing

Nursing has evolved into a profession with a distinct body of knowledge, university-based education, specialized practice, standards of practice, a social contract (ANA, 2010), and an ethical code (ANA, 2001). With this grounding, registered nurses and their profession are concerned with the availability and accessibility of nursing care to healthcare consumers, families, communities, and populations, and seek to ensure the integrity of nursing practice in all current and future healthcare systems. This professional evolution is described in the following pages.

Nursing Research and Evidence-Based Practice

Contemporary nursing practice has its historical roots in the poorhouses, the battlefields, and the industrial revolutions in nineteenth-century Europe and America. Initially nurses trained in hospital-based nursing schools and were employed mainly providing private care to patients in their homes. Florence Nightingale provided a foundation for nursing and the basis for autonomous nursing practice as distinct from medicine. Nightingale also is credited with identifying the importance of collecting empirical evidence, the underpinning of nursing's current emphasis on evidence-based practice, "What you want are facts, not opinions . . . The most important practical lesson that can be given to nurses is to teach them what to observe—how to observe—what symptoms indicate improvement—which are of none—which are the evidence of neglect— and what kind of neglect." (Nightingale, 1859, p. 105)

Although Nightingale recommended clinical nursing research in the mid-1800s, nurses did not follow her advice for over 100 years. Nursing research was able to flourish only as nurses received advanced educational preparation.

In the early 1900s nurses received their advanced degrees in nursing education, and thus nursing research was limited to studies of nurses and nursing education. However, case studies on nursing interventions were conducted in the 1920s and 1930s and the results published in the *American Journal of Nursing*.

In the 1950s, interest in nursing care studies began to rise. In 1952, the first issue of *Nursing Research* was published. In the 1960s, nursing studies began to explore theoretical and conceptual frameworks as a basis for practice. By the 1970s, more doctorally prepared nurses were conducting research, especially studies related to practice and the improvement of patient care. By the 1980s, there were greater numbers of qualified nurse researchers than ever before, and more computers available for collection and analysis of data. In 1985, the National Center for Nursing Research was established within the National Institutes of Health, putting nursing research into the mainstream of health research (Grant and Massey, 1999).

In the last half of the twentieth century, nurse researchers (1950s) and nurse theorists (1960s and 1970s) greatly contributed to the expanding body of nursing knowledge with their studies of nursing practice and the development of nursing models and theories. These conceptual models and theories borrow from other disciplines such as sociology, psychology, biology, and physics.

For example, the work of Neuman and King makes extensive use of systems theory. There is also Levine's conservation model, Roger's science of unitary human beings, Roy's adaptation model, Orem's self-care model, Peplau's interpersonal relations model, and Watson's theory of caring. The 1980s brought revisions to these theories, as well as additional theories developed by nursing leaders, such as Johnson, Parse, and Leininger, that added to the theoretical basis of nursing (George, 2002). In the 1990s, research tested and expanded these theories, which in turn continued to define and elaborate the discipline of nursing.

Evidence-based practice (EBP) is a scholarly and systematic problem-solving paradigm that results in the delivery of high-quality health care. In order to make the best clinical decisions using EBP, external evidence from research is blended with internal evidence (i.e., practice-generated data), clinical expertise, and healthcare consumer values and preferences to achieve the best outcomes for individuals, groups, populations, and healthcare systems.

Nursing's embrace of EBP is part of a larger call to integrate it into the entire spectrum of healthcare disciplines and professions. The Institute of Medicine (IOM) developed a vision for clinical education in the health professions that is centered on a commitment to meeting patient needs (IOM, 2003). This report

Appendix A. *Nursing: Scope and Standards of Practice, 2nd Edition (2010)*

The content in this appendix is not current and is of historical significance only.

stresses that all health disciplines must embrace evidence-based practice, quality improvement, and informatics in delivering healthcare consumer-centered care, and that their education should reflect and teach them to value those competencies. Interprofessional team collaboration is necessary to achieve quality outcomes for the improvement of health care.

Nursing research and EBP contribute to the body of knowledge and enhance outcomes. As a profession, nursing continually evaluates and applies nursing research findings. Evaluation of outcomes is a critical step in EBP. New knowledge is translated to healthcare consumer care to promote effective and efficient care and improved outcomes. It is then disseminated to decrease practice variations, improve outcomes, and create standards of excellence for care and policies. In addition, nurses ensure that changes in practice are based on current evidence; they should have expert resources in their practice environment and seek out those resources to assist them with specific steps in EBP.

The complex dynamics of health care, and demands for healthcare reform, will challenge the profession to quantify and qualify the value of nursing and nursing care. In alignment with the current edition of *Nursing's Social Policy Statement* (ANA, 2010) and this publication, the nursing profession continually examines nursing practice. An example is the study of unit-based nurse staffing levels, and demonstrating through evidence that safe staffing is imperative to quality patient care. This includes ongoing systematic evaluation of the impact of staffing and staffing effectiveness on patient outcomes.

Nursing's foundation as a profession took shape in the nineteenth century under Florence Nightingale, most notably with her work to provide quality nursing care for British soldiers during the Crimean War. But Nightingale also encouraged nurses to care for people beyond the sick bed, and to improve the health and safety of communities to promote wellness and prevent death (Nightingale, 1859). In the succeeding 150 years, nursing has expanded to almost every theater of health care.

Specialty Practice in Nursing

Nursing first expanded into public health interventions on behalf of at-risk communities and vulnerable populations. In 1893, Lillian Wald pioneered public health nursing at the Henry Street Settlement House in New York City. In 1899, Teacher's College at Columbia University offered the first university program for graduate nurses to specialize in public health nursing (Stewart, 1948). An editorial in the *American Journal of Nursing* in 1911 pointed out the urgent demand for nurses who could teach others and who could organize a whole community.

In the mid-twentieth century and beyond, advances in medical treatment and healthcare technology led to the evolution of other nursing specialties. Specialized education, training, and certification ensued in both traditional and newer areas of clinical practice, including medical-surgical nursing, pediatrics, anesthesia, midwifery, emergency care, mental health, public health, critical care, neonatal care, and primary care.

The continuation of the profession depends on the education of nurses, appropriate organization of nursing services, continued expansion of nursing knowledge, and the development and adoption of policies. Such initiatives demand that registered nurses be adequately prepared for these nursing specialties. Some specialties reflect the intersection of nursing's body of knowledge and that of another profession or discipline, directly influence nursing practice, and support the delivery of direct care rendered by registered nurses to healthcare consumers. Specialty nurses collaborate, consult, and serve as a liaison, bridging the role of the professional registered nurse with that of other professionals, and subsequently help to delineate nursing's role in society.

Registered nurses in specialty practice represent the full spectrum from novice to expert. Many nurses with an advanced graduate nursing education practice in specialties, such as informatics, public health, education, or administration, that are essential to advancing the public health but do not focus on direct care to individuals. Therefore, their practice does not require regulatory recognition beyond the Registered Nurse license granted by state boards of nursing.

Similarly, advanced practice registered nurses acquire specialized knowledge and skills through graduate-level education in their selected specialty areas. Competencies in individual specialty areas of practice are defined by separate specialty scope and standards documents, authored by specialty nursing associations. Many specialty nursing organizations recognize individual expertise through national certification in the specialty (see pages 92–94).

Advanced Practice Registered Nurse Roles

Another evolution of nursing practice was the development of educational programs to prepare nurses for advanced practice in direct care roles. These Advanced Practice Registered Nurse (APRN) roles include Certified Registered Nurse Anesthetists (CRNAs), Certified Nurse-Midwives (CNMs), Clinical

Appendix A. Nursing: Scope and Standards of Practice, 2nd Edition (2010)

Appendix A. *Nursing: Scope and Standards of Practice, 2nd Edition (2010)*

The content in this appendix is not current and is of historical significance only.

Nurse Specialists (CNSs), and Certified Nurse Practitioners (CNPs). Each has a unique history and context, but shares a focus on direct care to individual healthcare consumers.

Advanced Practice Registered Nurse is a regulatory title and includes the four roles listed above. The core competencies for education and the scope of practice are defined by the professional associations. State law and regulation further define criteria for licensure for the designated scopes of practice. The need to ensure healthcare consumer safety and access to APRNs by aligning education, accreditation, licensure, and certification is shown in *Consensus Model for APRN Regulation: Licensure, Accreditation, Certification, and Education* (APRN JDG, 2008).

In addition to the licensure, accreditation, certification, and education requirements for advanced practice registered nurses outlined in the Consensus Model, professional organizations have established standards and competencies for each advanced practice role:

- Accreditation Commission for Midwifery Education: *Criteria for Programmatic Accreditation* (2010)

- American Academy of Nurse Practitioners: *Standards of Practice for Nurse Practitioners* (2007)

- American Association of Nurse Anesthetists: *Scope and Standards for Nurse Anesthesia Practice* (2007)

- American College of Nurse-Midwives:

  - *Core Competencies for Basic Midwifery Practice* (2008)

  - *Standards for the Practice of Midwifery* (2009)

- Council on Accreditation of Nurse Anesthesia Educational Programs: *Competencies and Curricular Models* (2009)

- National Organization of Nurse Practitioner Faculties: *Domains and Core Competencies of Nurse Practitioner Practice* (2006)

- National Association of Clinical Nurse Specialists:

  - *Organizing Framework and CNS Core Competencies* (2008)

  - *Core Practice Doctorate Clinical Nurse Specialist (CNS) Competencies* (2009)

Nursing: Scope and Standards of Practice, 2nd Edition 19

Nurses in Advocacy and Society

Advocacy is a fundamental aspect of nursing practice. Registered nurses have long served as healthcare consumer advocates and used grassroots networking to influence social and political leaders and other advocates. Registered nurses firmly believe it is their obligation to help improve societal conditions related to healthcare consumer care, health, and wellness. Such issues have included protective labor laws, minimum wage, communicable disease programs, immunizations, well-baby and child care, women's health, curbing violence, reproductive health, end-of-life care, universal health care, social security, Medicare and Medicaid, the financing and reimbursement of health care, healthcare reform, ethics, mental health parity, confidentiality, workplace safety, and healthcare consumer rights.

There is ample need for professional nurses to continue advocacy and lobbying. These efforts include the evaluation and restructuring of health care, reimbursement and value of nursing care, funding for nursing education, the role of nursing in health and medical homes, comparative effectiveness, and advances in health information technology. Nurses will continue to remain strong advocates for healthcare consumers, their care, and health care.

The Progression of Nursing Education

ANA's long-held position is that the baccalaureate degree is the entry degree into nursing. But nursing's educational track to professional and career growth is not linear, and while there is an explicit progression of educational degrees, there is considerable flexibility in how the progression is achieved. Educational bodies are establishing entry-into-practice master's programs, associate's degree to baccalaureate or master's degree programs, and most notably second-degree baccalaureate programs.

Two new degrees have been introduced by the American Association of Colleges of Nursing (AACN) since 2004. The Doctor of Nursing Practice (DNP) was proposed as a generic clinical degree associated with practice-based nursing, and has been proposed by AACN to be the graduate degree for advanced nursing practice or specialty preparation by 2015 (AACN, 2004). The second degree is the Clinical Nurse Leader (CNL), described as an "advanced generalist" educated at the graduate level. A defining feature of the CNL role is an emphasis on health promotion, risk reduction, and population-based health care (AACN, 2008).

Appendix A. Nursing: Scope and Standards of Practice, 2nd Edition (2010)

IOM Influences on the Quality and Environment of Nursing Practice

To address issues in health care, the Institute of Medicine, a branch of the National Academy of Sciences, commissions reports on specific topics. While the IOM does not necessarily represent nursing, it does involve nurses in its work. Its reports and other publications are directed to universal medical practice, and sometimes explicitly to nursing, and provide a framework for systematic positive change in healthcare services.

In 1999, the Quality of Health Care in America Committee released the first and arguably most pivotal report, *To Err is Human: Building a Safer Health System*, which suggests that harm done to healthcare consumers in a profession that strives to "First, do no harm" is unacceptable. One of the most influential and paradigm-shifting conclusions of the report was that individuals and reckless behavior played only a small part in patient safety violations, and that faulty systems in which people were set up for failure were more problematic.

A second report by the committee in 2001, *Crossing the Quality Chasm: A New Health System for the 21st Century*, urges a fundamental, sweeping redesign of the entire health system. Incremental change was not enough. The committee suggested that such a system would not only improve patient safety and quality outcomes, but would also retain more health professionals who felt their contributions were making a satisfactory impact on those under their care.

Keeping Patients Safe: Transforming the Work Environment of Nurses is a key report for nurses; it considers how their interaction with their workplace helps or hinders patient care. The report reviews evidence on the work and work environments of nurses, and takes into account the behavioral traits of nurses, the organizational practices and culture, and the structural and engineering traits of the workplace. The report identifies components of the workplace most influential on nursing and patient outcomes—leadership and management, the workforce, work processes, and organizational culture—and proposes changes to these components that would lead to better outcomes for patients and nurses (IOM, 2004).

The connection between the nurse's work environment and patient mortality and failure to rescue was demonstrated by Aiken et al. (2008). Patients in hospitals with a better practice environment (characterized by nursing foundations for quality of care, nurse manager ability, leadership, and support, and collegial nurse–physician relations) fared far better than patients in hospitals with poor practice environments. To date, few work environments have achieved all of the IOM recommendations from 2004. The healthcare industry must alter the work environment of nurses to allow them to meet their social responsibility for healthcare consumer safety.

Integrating the Science and Art of Nursing

Nursing is a learned profession built on a core body of knowledge that reflects its dual components of science and art. Nursing requires judgment and skill based on principles of the biological, physical, behavioral, and social sciences. Nursing is a scientific discipline as well as a profession. Registered nurses employ critical thinking to integrate objective data with knowledge gained from an assessment of the subjective experiences of healthcare consumers. Registered nurses use critical thinking to apply the best available evidence and research data to diagnosis and treatment. Nurses continually evaluate quality and effectiveness of nursing practice and seek to optimize outcomes.

The Science of Nursing

The science of nursing is based on an analytical framework of critical thinking known as the nursing process, comprised of assessment, diagnosis, outcomes identification, planning, implementation, and evaluation. These steps serve as the foundation of clinical decision-making and support evidence-based practice. Wherever they practice, registered nurses use the nursing process and other types of critical thinking to respond to the needs of the populations they serve, and use strategies that support optimal outcomes most appropriate to the healthcare consumer or situation, being mindful of resource utilization.

Nurses as scientists rely on evidence to guide their policies and practices, but also as a way of quantifying the nurses' impact on the health outcomes of healthcare consumers. An example of ANA leadership in this area is the National Database of Nursing Quality Indicators (NDNQI®), a repository for nursing-sensitive indicators. NDNQI is the only database containing data collected at the nursing unit level.

The Art of Nursing

The art of nursing is based on caring and respect for human dignity. A compassionate approach to patient care carries a mandate to provide that care competently. Competent care is provided and accomplished through both independent practice and partnerships. Collaboration may be with other colleagues or with the individuals seeking support or assistance with their healthcare needs. Central to the nursing practice is the art of caring, which is represented in the personal relationship that the nurse enters with the patient. The art of caring goes beyond the emotional connections of humans to the ability to respond to the human aspects of health and illness within the critical moment to promote healing and calm (Watson 1999, 2008).

The art of nursing embraces dynamic processes that affect the human person, including, for example, spirituality, healing, empathy, mutual respect, and compassion. These intangible aspects foster health. Nursing embraces healing. Healing is fostered by compassion, helping, listening, mentoring, coaching, teaching, exploring, being present, supporting, touching, intuition, empathy, service, cultural competence, tolerance, acceptance, nurturing, mutually creating, and conflict resolution.

Nursing focuses on the promotion and maintenance of health and the prevention or resolution of disease, illness, or disability. The nursing needs of human beings are identified from a holistic perspective and are met in the context of a culturally sensitive, caring, personal relationship. Nursing includes the diagnosis and treatment of human responses to actual or potential health problems. Registered nurses employ practices that are restorative, supportive, and promotive in nature.

- *Restorative* practices modify the impact of illness or disease.

- *Supportive* practices are oriented toward modification of relationships or the practice environment to support health.

- *Promotive* practices mobilize healthy patterns of living, foster personal and family development, and support self-defined goals of individuals, families, communities, and populations.

Nursing's Societal and Ethical Dimensions

Nursing is responsive to the changing needs of society and the expanding knowledge base of its theoretical and scientific domains. One of nursing's objectives is to achieve positive healthcare consumer outcomes that maximize one's quality of life across the entire lifespan. Registered nurses facilitate the interprofessional and comprehensive care provided by healthcare professionals, paraprofessionals, and volunteers. In other instances, nurses engage in consultation with other colleagues to inform decision-making and planning to meet healthcare consumer needs. Registered nurses often participate in interprofessional teams in which the overlapping skills complement each member's individual efforts.

All nursing practice, regardless of specialty, role, or setting, is fundamentally independent practice. Registered nurses are accountable for nursing judgments made and actions taken in the course of their nursing practice. Therefore, the registered nurse is responsible for assessing individual competence and is committed to the process of lifelong learning. Registered nurses develop and maintain current knowledge and skills through formal and continuing education and seek certification when it is available in their areas of practice.

Registered nurses are bound by a professional code of ethics (ANA, 2001) and regulate themselves as individuals through a collegial process of peer review of practice. Peer evaluation fosters the refinement of knowledge, skills, and clinical decision-making at all levels and in all areas of clinical practice. Self-regulation by the profession of nursing assures quality of performance, which is the heart of nursing's social contract (ANA, 2010).

Registered nurses and members of various professions exchange knowledge and ideas about how to deliver high-quality health care, resulting in overlaps and constantly changing professional practice boundaries. This interprofessional team collaboration involves recognition of the expertise of others within and outside one's profession and referral to those providers when appropriate. Such collaboration also involves some shared functions and a common focus on one overall mission. By necessity, nursing's scope of practice has flexible boundaries.

Registered nurses regularly evaluate safety, effectiveness, and cost in the planning and delivery of nursing care. Nurses recognize that resources are limited and unequally distributed, and that the potential for better access to care requires innovative approaches, such as treating healthcare consumers remotely. As members of a profession, registered nurses work toward equitable distribution and availability of healthcare services throughout the nation and the world.

Caring and Nursing Practice

The essence of nursing practice is caring. "It is a beautiful and mysterious power that one human being can have on another through the mere act of caring . . . A great truth, the act of caring is the first step in the power to heal." (Moffitt, in *Relationship-Based Care*, 2004).

Watson (1999, 2008) emphasizes the personal relationship between patient and nurse. She highlights the role of the nurse in defining the patient as a unique human being and stresses the importance of the connections between the nurse and patient, modeled in her Transpersonal Caring-Healing Framework.

Leininger (1988) considers care for people from a broad range of cultures. Her five theoretical assumptions on caring are:

- Care is essential for human growth and survival, and to face death.

- There can be no curing without caring.

- Expressions of care vary among all cultures of the world.

- Therapeutic nursing care can only occur when cultural care values, expressions, or practices are known and used explicitly.

- Nursing is a transcultural care profession and discipline.

Swanson (1993) builds on Watson's framework and describes five caring processes and specific techniques for putting them into practice. The first two processes are internal processes of providing care; the other three are action processes.

- *Maintaining Belief*: Maintaining belief in persons and their capacity to make it through events and transitions

- *Knowing*: Striving to understand an event as it has meaning in the life of the other

- *Being With*: Being emotionally present to the other

Appendix A. Nursing: Scope and Standards of Practice, 2nd Edition (2010)

The content in this appendix is not current and is of historical significance only.

- *Doing For*: Doing for the other what they would do for themselves if it were possible

- *Enabling and Informing*: Facilitating the other's passage through life transitions and unfamiliar events

Continued Commitment to the Profession

A continued commitment to the nursing profession requires a nurse to remain involved in continuous learning and strengthening individual practice within varied practice settings. This may include civic activities, membership in and support of professional associations, collective bargaining, and workplace advocacy. The code of ethics (ANA, 2001) serves as the ethical framework in nursing regardless of practice setting or role, and provides guidance for the future.

Nurses promote the health of the individual and society regardless of cultural background, value system, religious belief, gender, sexual identity, or disability. Nurses commit to their profession by utilizing their skills, knowledge, and abilities to act as visionaries, promoting safe practice environments, and supporting resourceful, accessible, and cost-effective delivery of health care to serve the ever-changing needs of the population.

Professional Trends and Issues

Despite spending more on health care than any other nation, the United States ranks 42nd in the world in life expectancy (Trust for America's Health, 2009). A reformed healthcare system focused on primary care, prevention, and chronic disease management can alleviate the financial and social costs of treating preventable and chronic diseases. Interprofessional teams and coordination of care across the illness trajectory will be key components in the new system—arenas in which nurses are familiar and have demonstrated their value. Nurses at all levels are positioned to play key roles in a reformed and restructured care delivery system, such as:

- Coordinating healthcare consumers' transitions between healthcare delivery systems and settings (e.g., from hospital to rehabilitation to home)

- Monitoring and managing healthcare consumers with chronic disease

Appendix A. Nursing: Scope and Standards of Practice, 2nd Edition (2010)

- Promoting wellness and providing preventive health care
- Providing individualized care in nurse-managed health centers
- Participating in the "medical home" ("healthcare home") model for care management
- Utilizing advanced practice registered nurses to the fullest extent of their scope of practice consistent with education and competencies.

The nursing shortage looms as the greatest challenge to nurses to fill their critical role in health care. The aging nursing workforce, coupled with aging baby boomers, has created an imminent crisis in which record demand is timed to occur as nurses retire (Curtin, 2007). As more students are recruited into nursing, schools struggle to increase capacity. Faculty shortages—related to aging faculty, length of time to complete graduate education, heavy workload, and low salaries—severely hamper attempts by nursing schools to expand. Concern over the worsening shortage has provided the impetus for a number of innovative efforts to increase nursing capacity, including strategic partnerships to align and leverage stakeholder resources, increasing faculty capacity through accelerated programs and joint positions, redesigning nursing education, and changing policy and regulation (Joynt & Kimball, 2008).

In the face of healthcare reform and the nursing shortage, IOM and the Robert Wood Johnson Foundation have established a major initiative with the intent of "reconceptualizing the role of nurses within the context of the entire workforce, the shortage, societal issues, and current and future technology" (RWJF & IOM, 2009). The value of registered nurses in patient safety and positive patient outcomes in hospital settings is well demonstrated (Kane, Shamilyan, Mueller, Duval, & Wilt, 2007).

As healthcare reform evolves, nurses may experience greater opportunities to function within their full scope of practice across various settings. A reformed healthcare system will provide much needed incentives and financial support for utilizing nurses in various roles and promoting a full scope of practice, and eliminate the current payment practices that create barriers to innovative and effective models of practice and care delivery.

Employers are correcting workplace problems in an attempt to retain nurses. Safe patient handling, shift and scheduling options, integration of technology supports into practice, and alternative roles in the healthcare setting have enabled nurses to remain in the workplace.

Nursing: Scope and Standards of Practice, 2nd Edition 27

As the nurse of the future evolves, so must nursing education. Curricula must be designed to adequately prepare competent entry-level nurses. The nurse shortage and program capacity limits demand efficient educational processes. Online, virtual, simulated, and competency-based learning are attempts to expand opportunities to students and increase efficiency. However, design should be based on evidence more than tradition so that the nurse graduate is prepared to provide safe and competent care.

Nursing as a profession continues to face dilemmas in entry into practice, the autonomy of advanced practice, continued competence, multistate licensure, and the appropriate educational credentials for professional certification. Registered nurses have a professional responsibility to maintain competence in their area of practice. Employers who provide opportunities for professional development and continuing education promote a positive practice environment in which nurses can maintain and enhance skills and competencies.

Technology offers a better work environment for nurses when designed and implemented in a manner that supports nurses' work. These work environments can include conventional locations—hospitals, clinics, and healthcare consumer homes—as well as virtual spaces such as online discussion groups, email, interactive video, and virtual interaction. Ideally, technology eliminates redundancy and duplication of documentation; reduces errors; eliminates interruptions for missing supplies, equipment, and medications; and eases access to data, thereby allowing the nurse more time with the patient (Pamela Cipriano, PhD, RN, FAAN, in IOM, 2009). The incorporation of technologies, however, is not without risk, and demands diligence by registered nurses to consider the impact on the scope of nursing practice and the ethical implications for healthcare consumers as well as the nurse.

The healthcare industry has been challenged to improve patient safety, patient and practitioner satisfaction, patient outcomes, and the profitability of the healthcare organization (Kennedy, 2003). In 1999 IOM described the nation's healthcare system as fractured, prone to errors, and detrimental to safe patient care. IOM has identified six aims for improvement so that the healthcare system is: safe, effective, patient-centered, timely, efficient, and equitable (IOM, 2001).

Whatever the practice venue, in the next decade registered nurses will continue to partner with others to advance the nation's health through many initiatives, such as *Healthy People 2020*. Such partnerships truly reflect the definition of nursing and illustrate the essential features of contemporary nursing practice:

- A caring relationship that facilitates health and healing

- Attention to the range of human experiences and responses to health, disease, and illness in the physical and social environments

- Integration of objective data with knowledge gained from an appreciation of the healthcare consumer's or group's subjective experience

- Application of scientific knowledge to diagnosis and treatment through the use of judgment and critical thinking

- Advancement of professional nursing knowledge through scholarly inquiry

- Influence on social and public policy to promote social justice (ANA, 2010)

Summary of the Scope of Nursing Practice

The dynamic nature of the healthcare practice environment and the growing body of nursing research provide both the impetus and the opportunity for nursing to ensure competent nursing practice in all settings for all healthcare consumers and to promote ongoing professional development that enhances the quality of nursing practice. *Nursing: Scope and Standards of Practice, Second Edition*, assists that process by delineating the professional scope and standards of practice and responsibilities of all professional registered nurses engaged in nursing practice, regardless of setting. As such, it can serve as a basis for:

- Quality improvement systems

- Regulatory systems

- Healthcare reimbursement and financing methodologies

- Development and evaluation of nursing service delivery systems and organizational structures

- Certification activities

- Position descriptions and performance appraisals
- Agency policies, procedures, and protocols
- Educational offerings
- Establishing the legal standard of care

To best serve the public's health and the nursing profession, nursing must continue its efforts to establish the Standards of Professional Nursing Practice. Nursing also must examine how the Standards of Professional Nursing Practice can be disseminated and used most effectively to enhance and promote the quality of practice. In addition, the Standards of Professional Nursing Practice must be continually evaluated and revised as necessary.

The dynamic healthcare practice environment and the growing body of nursing research provide both the impetus and the opportunity for nursing to ensure competent nursing practice in all settings for all healthcare consumers and to promote ongoing professional development that enhances the quality of nursing practice.

Standards of Professional Nursing Practice

Significance of Standards

The Standards of Professional Nursing Practice are authoritative statements of the duties that all registered nurses, regardless of role, population, or specialty, are expected to perform competently. The standards published herein may be utilized as evidence of the standard of care, with the understanding that application of the standards is context dependent. The standards are subject to change with the dynamics of the nursing profession, as new patterns of professional practice are developed and accepted by the nursing profession and the public. In addition, specific conditions and clinical circumstances may also affect the application of the standards at a given time, e.g., during a natural disaster. The standards are subject to formal, periodic review and revision. (See page 87 for information of this review and revision process.)

The Standards of Professional Nursing Practice are authoritative statements of the duties that all registered nurses, regardless of role, population, or specialty, are expected to perform competently. The standards published herein:

- May be utilized as evidence of the standard of care, with the understanding that application of the standards is context dependent

- Are subject to change with the dynamics of the nursing profession, as new patterns of professional practice are developed and accepted by the nursing profession and the public, and

- Are subject to formal, periodic review and revision.

The competencies that accompany each standard may be evidence of compliance with the corresponding standard. The list of competencies is not exhaustive for a given standard. Whether a particular standard or competency applies depends upon the circumstances.

31

Standards of Practice

Standard 1. Assessment

The registered nurse collects comprehensive data pertinent to the healthcare consumer's health and/or the situation.

COMPETENCIES

The registered nurse:

- Collects comprehensive data including but not limited to physical, functional, psychosocial, emotional, cognitive, sexual, cultural, age-related, environmental, spiritual/transpersonal, and economic assessments in a systematic and ongoing process while honoring the uniqueness of the person.

- Elicits the healthcare consumer's values, preferences, expressed needs, and knowledge of the healthcare situation.

- Involves the healthcare consumer, family, and other healthcare providers as appropriate, in holistic data collection.

- Identifies barriers (e.g., psychosocial, literacy, financial, cultural) to effective communication and makes appropriate adaptations.

- Recognizes the impact of personal attitudes, values, and beliefs.

- Assesses family dynamics and impact on healthcare consumer health and wellness.

- Prioritizes data collection based on the healthcare consumer's immediate condition, or the anticipated needs of the healthcare consumer or situation.

- Uses appropriate evidence-based assessment techniques, instruments, and tools.

- Synthesizes available data, information, and knowledge relevant to the situation to identify patterns and variances.

- Applies ethical, legal, and privacy guidelines and policies to the collection, maintenance, use, and dissemination of data and information.
- Recognizes the healthcare consumer as the authority on her or his own health by honoring their care preferences.
- Documents relevant data in a retrievable format.

ADDITIONAL COMPETENCIES FOR THE GRADUATE-LEVEL PREPARED SPECIALTY NURSE AND THE APRN

The graduate-level prepared specialty nurse or the advanced practice registered nurse:

- Initiates and interprets diagnostic tests and procedures relevant to the healthcare consumer's current status.
- Assesses the effect of interactions among individuals, family, community, and social systems on health and illness.

Standard 2. Diagnosis

The registered nurse analyzes the assessment data to determine the diagnoses or the issues.

COMPETENCIES

The registered nurse:

- Derives the diagnoses or issues from assessment data.

- Validates the diagnoses or issues with the healthcare consumer, family, and other healthcare providers when possible and appropriate.

- Identifies actual or potential risks to the healthcare consumer's health and safety or barriers to health, which may include but are not limited to interpersonal, systematic, or environmental circumstances.

- Uses standardized classification systems and clinical decision support tools, when available, in identifying diagnoses.

- Documents diagnoses or issues in a manner that facilitates the determination of the expected outcomes and plan.

ADDITIONAL COMPETENCIES FOR THE GRADUATE-LEVEL PREPARED SPECIALTY NURSE AND THE APRN

The graduate-level prepared specialty nurse or the advanced practice registered nurse:

- Systematically compares and contrasts clinical findings with normal and abnormal variations and developmental events in formulating a differential diagnosis.

- Utilizes complex data and information obtained during interview, examination, and diagnostic processes in identifying diagnoses.

- Assists staff in developing and maintaining competency in the diagnostic process.

Appendix A. Nursing: Scope and Standards of Practice, 2nd Edition (2010)

Standard 3. Outcomes Identification

The registered nurse identifies expected outcomes for a plan individualized to the healthcare consumer or the situation.

COMPETENCIES

The registered nurse:

- Involves the healthcare consumer, family, healthcare providers, and others in formulating expected outcomes when possible and appropriate.

- Derives culturally appropriate expected outcomes from the diagnoses.

- Considers associated risks, benefits, costs, current scientific evidence, expected trajectory of the condition, and clinical expertise when formulating expected outcomes.

- Defines expected outcomes in terms of the healthcare consumer, healthcare consumer culture, values, and ethical considerations.

- Includes a time estimate for the attainment of expected outcomes.

- Develops expected outcomes that facilitate continuity of care.

- Modifies expected outcomes according to changes in the status of the healthcare consumer or evaluation of the situation.

- Documents expected outcomes as measurable goals.

ADDITIONAL COMPETENCIES FOR THE GRADUATE-LEVEL PREPARED SPECIALTY NURSE AND THE APRN

The graduate-level prepared specialty nurse or the advanced practice registered nurse:

- Identifies expected outcomes that incorporate scientific evidence and are achievable through implementation of evidence-based practices.

- Identifies expected outcomes that incorporate cost and clinical effectiveness, healthcare consumer satisfaction, and continuity and consistency among providers.

- Differentiates outcomes that require care process interventions from those that require system-level interventions.

Standard 4. Planning

The registered nurse develops a plan that prescribes strategies and alternatives to attain expected outcomes.

COMPETENCIES

The registered nurse:

- Develops an individualized plan in partnership with the person, family, and others considering the person's characteristics or situation, including, but not limited to, values, beliefs, spiritual and health practices, preferences, choices, developmental level, coping style, culture and environment, and available technology.

- Establishes the plan priorities with the healthcare consumer, family, and others as appropriate.

- Includes strategies in the plan that address each of the identified diagnoses or issues. These may include, but are not limited to, strategies for:

  - Promotion and restoration of health;

  - Prevention of illness, injury, and disease;

  - The alleviation of suffering; and

  - Supportive care for those who are dying.

- Includes strategies for health and wholeness across the lifespan.

- Provides for continuity in the plan.

- Incorporates an implementation pathway or timeline in the plan.

- Considers the economic impact of the plan on the healthcare consumer, family, caregivers, or other affected parties.

- Integrates current scientific evidence, trends and research.

- Utilizes the plan to provide direction to other members of the healthcare team.

Appendix A. Nursing: Scope and Standards of Practice, 2nd Edition (2010)

■ Explores practice settings and safe space and time for the nurse and the healthcare consumer to explore suggested, potential, and alternative options.

■ Defines the plan to reflect current statutes, rules and regulations, and standards.

■ Modifies the plan according to the ongoing assessment of the healthcare consumer's response and other outcome indicators.

■ Documents the plan in a manner that uses standardized language or recognized terminology.

ADDITIONAL COMPETENCIES FOR THE GRADUATE-LEVEL PREPARED SPECIALTY NURSE AND THE APRN

The graduate-level prepared specialty nurse or the advanced practice registered nurse:

■ Identifies assessment strategies, diagnostic strategies, and therapeutic interventions that reflect current evidence, including data, research, literature, and expert clinical knowledge.

■ Selects or designs strategies to meet the multifaceted needs of complex healthcare consumers.

■ Includes the synthesis of healthcare consumers' values and beliefs regarding nursing and medical therapies in the plan.

■ Leads the design and development of interprofessional processes to address the identified diagnosis or issue.

■ Actively participates in the development and continuous improvement of systems that support the planning process.

Nursing: Scope and Standards of Practice, 2nd Edition 37

Standard 5. Implementation

The registered nurse implements the identified plan.

COMPETENCIES

The registered nurse:

- Partners with the person, family, significant others, and caregivers as appropriate to implement the plan in a safe, realistic, and timely manner.

- Demonstrates caring behaviors toward healthcare consumers, significant others, and groups of people receiving care.

- Utilizes technology to measure, record, and retrieve healthcare consumer data, implement the nursing process, and enhance nursing practice

- Utilizes evidence-based interventions and treatments specific to the diagnosis or problem.

- Provides holistic care that addresses the needs of diverse populations across the lifespan.

- Advocates for health care that is sensitive to the needs of healthcare consumers, with particular emphasis on the needs of diverse populations.

- Applies appropriate knowledge of major health problems and cultural diversity in implementing the plan of care.

- Applies available healthcare technologies to maximize access and optimize outcomes for healthcare consumers.

- Utilizes community resources and systems to implement the plan.

- Collaborates with healthcare providers from diverse backgrounds to implement and integrate the plan.

- Accommodates for different styles of communication used by healthcare consumers, families, and healthcare providers.

- Integrates traditional and complementary healthcare practices as appropriate.

Appendix A. Nursing: Scope and Standards of Practice, 2nd Edition (2010)

- Implements the plan in a timely manner in accordance with patient safety goals.

- Promotes the healthcare consumer's capacity for the optimal level of participation and problem-solving.

- Documents implementation and any modifications, including changes or omissions, of the identified plan

ADDITIONAL COMPETENCIES FOR THE GRADUATE-LEVEL PREPARED SPECIALTY NURSE AND THE APRN

The graduate-level prepared specialty nurse or the advanced practice registered nurse:

- Facilitates utilization of systems, organizations, and community resources to implement the plan.

- Supports collaboration with nursing and other colleagues to implement the plan.

- Incorporates new knowledge and strategies to initiate change in nursing care practices if desired outcomes are not achieved.

- Assumes responsibility for the safe and efficient implementation of the plan.

- Use advanced communication skills to promote relationships between nurses and healthcare consumers, to provide a context for open discussion of the healthcare consumer's experiences, and to improve healthcare consumer outcomes.

- Actively participates in the development and continuous improvement of systems that support the implementation of the plan.

Appendix A. *Nursing: Scope and Standards of Practice, 2nd Edition (2010)*

Standard 5A. Coordination of Care

The registered nurse coordinates care delivery.

COMPETENCIES

The registered nurse:

- Organizes the components of the plan.

- Manages a healthcare consumer's care in order to maximize independence and quality of life.

- Assists the healthcare consumer in identifying options for alternative care.

- Communicates with the healthcare consumer, family, and system during transitions in care.

- Advocates for the delivery of dignified and humane care by the interprofessional team.

- Documents the coordination of care.

ADDITIONAL COMPETENCIES FOR THE GRADUATE-LEVEL PREPARED SPECIALTY NURSE AND THE APRN

The graduate-level prepared specialty nurse or the advanced practice registered nurse:

- Provides leadership in the coordination of interprofessional health care for integrated delivery of healthcare consumer care services.

- Synthesizes data and information to prescribe necessary system and community support measures, including modifications of surroundings.

Standard 5B. Health Teaching and Health Promotion

The registered nurse employs strategies to promote health and a safe environment.

COMPETENCIES

The registered nurse:

- Provides health teaching that addresses such topics as healthy lifestyles, risk-reducing behaviors, developmental needs, activities of daily living, and preventive self-care.

- Uses health promotion and health teaching methods appropriate to the situation and the healthcare consumer's values, beliefs, health practices, developmental level, learning needs, readiness and ability to learn, language preference, spirituality, culture, and socioeconomic status.

- Seeks opportunities for feedback and evaluation of the effectiveness of the strategies used.

- Uses information technologies to communicate health promotion and disease prevention information to the healthcare consumer in a variety of settings.

- Provides healthcare consumers with information about intended effects and potential adverse effects of proposed therapies.

ADDITIONAL COMPETENCIES FOR THE GRADUATE-LEVEL PREPARED SPECIALTY NURSE AND THE APRN

The graduate-level prepared specialty nurse or the advanced practice registered nurse:

- Synthesizes empirical evidence on risk behaviors, learning theories, behavioral change theories, motivational theories, epidemiology, and other related theories and frameworks when designing health education information and programs.

- Conducts personalized health teaching and counseling considering comparative effectiveness research recommendations.

Continued ▶

- Designs health information and healthcare consumer education appropriate to the healthcare consumer's developmental level, learning needs, readiness to learn, and cultural values and beliefs.

- Evaluates health information resources, such as the Internet, in the area of practice for accuracy, readability, and comprehensibility to help healthcare consumers access quality health information.

- Engages consumer alliances and advocacy groups, as appropriate, in health teaching and health promotion activities.

- Provides anticipatory guidance to individuals, families, groups, and communities to promote health and prevent or reduce the risk of health problems.

Appendix A. Nursing: Scope and Standards of Practice, 2nd Edition (2010)

Standard 5C. Consultation

The graduate-level prepared specialty nurse or advanced practice registered nurse provides consultation to influence the identified plan, enhance the abilities of others, and effect change.

COMPETENCIES FOR THE GRADUATE-LEVEL PREPARED SPECIALTY NURSE AND THE APRN

The graduate-level prepared specialty nurse or the advanced practice registered nurse:

- Synthesizes clinical data, theoretical frameworks, and evidence when providing consultation.

- Facilitates the effectiveness of a consultation by involving the health-care consumers and stakeholders in decision-making and negotiating role responsibilities.

- Communicates consultation recommendations.

Standard 5D. Prescriptive Authority and Treatment

The advanced practice registered nurse uses prescriptive authority, procedures, referrals, treatments, and therapies in accordance with state and federal laws and regulations.

COMPETENCIES FOR THE ADVANCED PRACTICE REGISTERED NURSE

The advanced practice registered nurse:

- Prescribes evidence-based treatments, therapies, and procedures considering the healthcare consumer's comprehensive healthcare needs.

- Prescribes pharmacologic agents based on a current knowledge of pharmacology and physiology.

- Prescribes specific pharmacological agents or treatments according to clinical indicators, the healthcare consumer's status and needs, and the results of diagnostic and laboratory tests.

- Evaluates therapeutic and potential adverse effects of pharmacological and nonpharmacological treatments.

- Provides healthcare consumers with information about intended effects and potential adverse effects of proposed prescriptive therapies.

- Provides information about costs and alternative treatments and procedures, as appropriate.

- Evaluates and incorporates complementary and alternative therapy into education and practice.

Appendix A. *Nursing: Scope and Standards of Practice, 2nd Edition (2010)*

Standard 6. Evaluation

The registered nurse evaluates progress toward attainment of outcomes.

COMPETENCIES

The registered nurse:

- Conducts a systematic, ongoing, and criterion-based evaluation of the outcomes in relation to the structures and processes prescribed by the plan of care and the indicated timeline.

- Collaborates with the healthcare consumer and others involved in the care or situation in the evaluation process.

- Evaluates, in partnership with the healthcare consumer, the effectiveness of the planned strategies in relation to the healthcare consumer's responses and the attainment of the expected outcomes.

- Uses ongoing assessment data to revise the diagnoses, outcomes, the plan, and the implementation as needed.

- Disseminates the results to the healthcare consumer, family, and others involved, in accordance with federal and state regulations.

- Participates in assessing and assuring the responsible and appropriate use of interventions in order to minimize unwarranted or unwanted treatment and healthcare consumer suffering.

- Documents the results of the evaluation.

ADDITIONAL COMPETENCIES FOR THE GRADUATE-LEVEL PREPARED SPECIALTY NURSE AND THE APRN

The graduate-level prepared specialty nurse or the advanced practice registered nurse:

- Evaluates the accuracy of the diagnosis and the effectiveness of the interventions and other variables in relation to the healthcare consumer's attainment of expected outcomes.

Continued ▶

- Synthesizes the results of the evaluation to determine the effect of the plan on healthcare consumers, families, groups, communities, and institutions.

- Adapts the plan of care for the trajectory of treatment according to evaluation of response.

- Uses the results of the evaluation to make or recommend process or structural changes including policy, procedure, or protocol revision, as appropriate.

Standards of Professional Performance

Standard 7. Ethics

The registered nurse practices ethically.

COMPETENCIES

The registered nurse:

- Uses *Code of Ethics for Nurses with Interpretive Statements* (ANA, 2001) to guide practice.

- Delivers care in a manner that preserves and protects healthcare consumer autonomy, dignity, rights, values, and beliefs.

- Recognizes the centrality of the healthcare consumer and family as core members of any healthcare team.

- Upholds healthcare consumer confidentiality within legal and regulatory parameters.

- Assists healthcare consumers in self determination and informed decision-making.

- Maintains a therapeutic and professional healthcare consumer–nurse relationship within appropriate professional role boundaries.

- Contributes to resolving ethical issues involving healthcare consumers, colleagues, community groups, systems, and other stakeholders.

- Takes appropriate action regarding instances of illegal, unethical, or inappropriate behavior that can endanger or jeopardize the best interests of the healthcare consumer or situation.

- Speaks up when appropriate to question healthcare practice when necessary for safety and quality improvement.

- Advocates for equitable healthcare consumer care.

Continued ▶

ADDITIONAL COMPETENCIES FOR THE GRADUATE-LEVEL PREPARED SPECIALTY NURSE AND THE APRN

The graduate-level prepared specialty nurse or the advanced practice registered nurse:

- Participates in interprofessional teams that address ethical risks, benefits, and outcomes.

- Provides information on the risks, benefits, and outcomes of healthcare regimens to allow informed decision-making by the healthcare consumer, including informed consent and informed refusal.

Appendix A. Nursing: Scope and Standards of Practice, 2nd Edition (2010)

Standard 8. Education

The registered nurse attains knowledge and competence that reflects current nursing practice.

COMPETENCIES

The registered nurse:

- Participates in ongoing educational activities related to appropriate knowledge bases and professional issues.

- Demonstrates a commitment to lifelong learning through self-reflection and inquiry to address learning and personal growth needs.

- Seeks experiences that reflect current practice to maintain knowledge, skills, abilities, and judgment in clinical practice or role performance.

- Acquires knowledge and skills appropriate to the role, population, specialty, setting, role, or situation.

- Seeks formal and independent learning experiences to develop and maintain clinical and professional skills and knowledge.

- Identifies learning needs based on nursing knowledge, the various roles the nurse may assume, and the changing needs of the population.

- Participates in formal or informal consultations to address issues in nursing practice as an application of education and a knowledge base.

- Shares educational findings, experiences, and ideas with peers.

- Contributes to a work environment conducive to the education of healthcare professionals.

- Maintains professional records that provide evidence of competence and lifelong learning.

Continued ▶

ADDITIONAL COMPETENCIES FOR THE GRADUATE-LEVEL PREPARED SPECIALTY NURSE AND THE APRN

The graduate-level prepared specialty nurse or the advanced practice registered nurse:

- Uses current healthcare research findings and other evidence to expand clinical knowledge, skills, abilities, and judgment, to enhance role performance, and to increase knowledge of professional issues.

Appendix A. Nursing: Scope and Standards of Practice, 2nd Edition (2010)

Standard 9. Evidence-Based Practice and Research

The registered nurse integrates evidence and research findings into practice.

COMPETENCIES

The registered nurse:

- Utilizes current evidence-based nursing knowledge, including research findings, to guide practice.

- Incorporates evidence when initiating changes in nursing practice.

- Participates, as appropriate to education level and position, in the formulation of evidence-based practice through research.

- Shares personal or third-party research findings with colleagues and peers.

ADDITIONAL COMPETENCIES FOR THE GRADUATE-LEVEL PREPARED SPECIALTY NURSE AND THE APRN

The graduate-level prepared specialty nurse or the advanced practice registered nurse:

- Contributes to nursing knowledge by conducting or synthesizing research and other evidence that discovers, examines, and evaluates current practice, knowledge, theories, criteria, and creative approaches to improve healthcare outcomes.

- Promotes a climate of research and clinical inquiry.

- Disseminates research findings through activities such as presentations, publications, consultation, and journal clubs.

Standard 10. Quality of Practice

The registered nurse contributes to quality nursing practice.

COMPETENCIES

The registered nurse:

- Demonstrates quality by documenting the application of the nursing process in a responsible, accountable, and ethical manner.

- Uses creativity and innovation to enhance nursing care.

- Participates in quality improvement. Activities may include:

  - Identifying aspects of practice important for quality monitoring;

  - Using indicators to monitor quality, safety, and effectiveness of nursing practice;

  - Collecting data to monitor quality and effectiveness of nursing practice;

  - Analyzing quality data to identify opportunities for improving nursing practice;

  - Formulating recommendations to improve nursing practice or outcomes;

  - Implementing activities to enhance the quality of nursing practice;

  - Developing, implementing, and/or evaluating policies, procedures, and guidelines to improve the quality of practice;

  - Participating on and/or leading interprofessional teams to evaluate clinical care or health services;

  - Participating in and/or leading efforts to minimize costs and unnecessary duplication;

  - Identifying problems that occur in day-to-day work routines in order to correct process inefficiencies;*

  - Analyzing factors related to quality, safety, and effectiveness,

---

*BHE/MONE, 2006.

- Analyzing organizational systems for barriers to quality healthcare consumer outcomes; and

- Implementing processes to remove or weaken barriers within organizational systems.

ADDITIONAL COMPETENCIES FOR THE GRADUATE-LEVEL PREPARED SPECIALTY NURSE AND THE APRN

The graduate-level prepared specialty nurse or the advanced practice registered nurse:

- Provides leadership in the design and implementation of quality improvements.

- Designs innovations to effect change in practice and improve health outcomes.

- Evaluates the practice environment and quality of nursing care rendered in relation to existing evidence.

- Identifies opportunities for the generation and use of research and evidence.

- Obtains and maintains professional certification if it is available in the area of expertise.

- Uses the results of quality improvement to initiate changes in nursing practice and the healthcare delivery system.

Standard 11. Communication

The registered nurse communicates effectively in a variety of formats in all areas of practice.

COMPETENCIES

The registered nurse:

- Assesses communication format preferences of healthcare consumers, families, and colleagues.*

- Assesses her or his own communication skills in encounters with healthcare consumers, families, and colleagues.*

- Seeks continuous improvement of communication and conflict resolution skills.*

- Conveys information to healthcare consumers, families, the interprofessional team, and others in communication formats that promote accuracy.

- Questions the rationale supporting care processes and decisions when they do not appear to be in the best interest of the patient.*

- Discloses observations or concerns related to hazards and errors in care or the practice environment to the appropriate level.

- Maintains communication with other providers to minimize risks associated with transfers and transition in care delivery.

- Contributes her or his own professional perspective in discussions with the interprofessional team.

*BHE/MONE, 2006.

Standard 12. Leadership

The registered nurse demonstrates leadership in the professional practice setting and the profession.

COMPETENCIES

The registered nurse:

- Oversees the nursing care given by others while retaining accountability for the quality of care given to the healthcare consumer.

- Abides by the vision, the associated goals, and the plan to implement and measure progress of an individual healthcare consumer or progress within the context of the healthcare organization.

- Demonstrates a commitment to continuous, lifelong learning and education for self and others.

- Mentors colleagues for the advancement of nursing practice, the profession, and quality health care.

- Treats colleagues with respect, trust, and dignity.*

- Develops communication and conflict resolution skills.

- Participates in professional organizations.

- Communicates effectively with the healthcare consumer and colleagues.

- Seeks ways to advance nursing autonomy and accountability.*

- Participates in efforts to influence healthcare policy involving healthcare consumers and the profession.*

---

*BHE/MONE, 2006.

Continued ▶

Nursing: Scope and Standards of Practice, 2nd Edition   55

ADDITIONAL COMPETENCIES FOR THE GRADUATE-LEVEL PREPARED SPECIALTY NURSE AND THE APRN

The graduate-level prepared specialty nurse or the advanced practice registered nurse:

- Influences decision-making bodies to improve the professional practice environment and healthcare consumer outcomes.

- Provides direction to enhance the effectiveness of the interprofessional team.

- Promotes advanced practice nursing and role development by interpreting its role for healthcare consumers, families, and others.

- Models expert practice to interprofessional team members and healthcare consumers.

- Mentors colleagues in the acquisition of clinical knowledge, skills, abilities, and judgment.

Appendix A. Nursing: Scope and Standards of Practice, 2nd Edition (2010)

Appendix A. *Nursing: Scope and Standards of Practice, 2nd Edition (2010)*

Standard 13. Collaboration

The registered nurse collaborates with healthcare consumer, family, and others in the conduct of nursing practice.

COMPETENCIES

The registered nurse:

- Partners with others to effect change and produce positive outcomes through the sharing of knowledge of the healthcare consumer and/or situation.

- Communicates with the healthcare consumer, the family, and health-care providers regarding healthcare consumer care and the nurse's role in the provision of that care.

- Promotes conflict management and engagement.

- Participates in building consensus or resolving conflict in the context of patient care.

- Applies group process and negotiation techniques with healthcare consumers and colleagues.

- Adheres to standards and applicable codes of conduct that govern behavior among peers and colleagues to create a work environment that promotes cooperation, respect, and trust.

- Cooperates in creating a documented plan focused on outcomes and decisions related to care and delivery of services that indicates communication with healthcare consumers, families, and others.

- Engages in teamwork and team-building process.

Continued ▶

Nursing: Scope and Standards of Practice, 2nd Edition 57

ADDITIONAL COMPETENCIES FOR THE GRADUATE-LEVEL PREPARED SPECIALTY NURSE AND THE APRN

The graduate-level prepared specialty nurse or the advanced practice registered nurse:

- Partners with other disciplines to enhance healthcare consumer outcomes through interprofessional activities, such as education, consultation, management, technological development, or research opportunities.

- Invites the contribution of the healthcare consumer, family, and team members in order to achieved optimal outcomes.

- Leads in establishing, improving, and sustaining collaborative relationships to achieve safe, quality healthcare consumer care.

- Documents plan-of-care communications, rationales for plan-of-care changes, and collaborative discussions to improve healthcare consumer outcomes.

Standard 14. Professional Practice Evaluation

The registered nurse evaluates her or his own nursing practice in relation to professional practice standards and guidelines, relevant statutes, rules, and regulations.

COMPETENCIES

The registered nurse:

- Provides age-appropriate and developmentally appropriate care in a culturally and ethnically sensitive manner.

- Engages in self-evaluation of practice on a regular basis, identifying areas of strength as well as areas in which professional growth would be beneficial.

- Obtains informal feedback regarding her or his own practice from healthcare consumers, peers, professional colleagues, and others.

- Participates in peer review as appropriate.

- Takes action to achieve goals identified during the evaluation process.

- Provides the evidence for practice decisions and actions as part of the informal and formal evaluation processes.

- Interacts with peers and colleagues to enhance her or his own professional nursing practice or role performance.

- Provides peers with formal or informal constructive feedback regarding their practice or role performance.

ADDITIONAL COMPETENCIES FOR THE GRADUATE-LEVEL PREPARED SPECIALTY NURSE AND THE APRN

The graduate-level prepared specialty nurse or the advanced practice registered nurse:

- Engages in a formal process seeking feedback regarding her or his own practice from healthcare consumers, peers, professional colleagues, and others.

Nursing: Scope and Standards of Practice, 2nd Edition   59

Standard 15. Resource Utilization

The registered nurse utilizes appropriate resources to plan and provide nursing services that are safe, effective, and financially responsible.

COMPETENCIES

The registered nurse:

- Assesses individual healthcare consumer care needs and resources available to achieve desired outcomes.

- Identifies healthcare consumer care needs, potential for harm, complexity of the task, and desired outcome when considering resource allocation.

- Delegates elements of care to appropriate healthcare workers in accordance with any applicable legal or policy parameters or principles.

- Identifies the evidence when evaluating resources.

- Advocates for resources, including technology, that enhance nursing practice.

- Modifies practice when necessary to promote positive interaction between healthcare consumers, care providers, and technology.

- Assists the healthcare consumer and family in identifying and securing appropriate services to address needs across the healthcare continuum.

- Assists the healthcare consumer and family in factoring costs, risks, and benefits in decisions about treatment and care.

ADDITIONAL COMPETENCIES FOR THE GRADUATE-LEVEL PREPARED SPECIALTY NURSE AND THE APRN

The graduate-level prepared specialty nurse or the advanced practice registered nurse:

- Utilizes organizational and community resources to formulate inter-professional plans of care.

- Formulates innovative solutions for healthcare consumer care problems that utilize resources effectively and maintain quality.

- Designs evaluation strategies that demonstrate cost-effectiveness, cost-benefit, and efficiency factors associated with nursing practice.

Appendix A. *Nursing: Scope and Standards of Practice, 2nd Edition (2010)*

Standard 16. Environmental Health

The registered nurse practices in an environmentally safe and healthy manner.

COMPETENCIES

The registered nurse:

- Attains knowledge of environmental health concepts, such as implementation of environmental health strategies.

- Promotes a practice environment that reduces environmental health risks for workers and healthcare consumers.

- Assesses the practice environment for factors such as sound, odor, noise, and light that threaten health.

- Advocates for the judicious and appropriate use of products in health care.

- Communicates environmental health risks and exposure reduction strategies to healthcare consumers, families, colleagues, and communities.

- Utilizes scientific evidence to determine if a product or treatment is an environmental threat.

- Participates in strategies to promote healthy communities.

ADDITIONAL COMPETENCIES FOR THE GRADUATE-LEVEL PREPARED SPECIALTY NURSE AND THE APRN

The graduate-level prepared specialty nurse or the advanced practice registered nurse:

- Creates partnerships that promote sustainable environmental health policies and conditions.

- Analyzes the impact of social, political, and economic influences on the environment and human health exposures.

Continued ▶

- Critically evaluates the manner in which environmental health issues are presented by the popular media.

- Advocates for implementation of environmental principles for nursing practice.

- Supports nurses in advocating for and implementing environmental principles in nursing practice.

Appendix A. Nursing: Scope and Standards of Practice, 2nd Edition (2010)

References and Bibliography

All URLs were retrieved on August 18, 2010.

Accreditation Commission for Midwifery Education (ACME). (2010). *Criteria for programmatic accreditation.* Silver Spring: Author. http://www.midwife.org/acmedocs/ACME.Programmatic.Criteria .Final.June.2010.pdf

American Academy of Nurse Practitioners (AANP). (2007). *Standards of practice for nurse practitioners.* Washington, DC: Author. http:// www.aanp.org/NR/rdonlyres/FE00E81B-FA96-4779-972B-6162F04C309F/0/Standards_of_Practice112907.pdf

American Association of Colleges of Nursing (AACN). (2004). *AACN position statement on the practice doctorate in nursing.* October 2004 Washington, DC: Author.

American Association of Colleges of Nursing (AACN). (2008). *The essentials of baccalaureate education for professional nursing practice.* Washington, DC: Author.

American Association of Critical-Care Nurses (AACN). (2005). *AACN standards for establishing and maintaining healthy work environments.* Mission Viejo, CA: Author.

69

American Association of Nurse Anesthetists (AANA). Council on Accreditation of Nurse Anesthesia Educational Programs (COA). (n.d). *Competencies and curricular models.* Park Ridge, IL: Author. http://www.aana.com/uploadedFiles/Professional_Development/ Nurse_Anesthesia_Education/Educational_Resources/DTF_Report/ competencies.pdf

American Association of Nurse Anesthetists (AANA). (2007). *Scope and standards for nurse anesthesia practice.* Park Ridge, IL: Author. http://www.aana.com/uploadedFiles/Resources/Practice_Documents/ scope_stds_nap07_2007.pdf

American College of Nurse-Midwives (ACNM). (2008). *Core competencies for basic midwifery practice.* Silver Spring: Author. http://www.midwife. org/siteFiles/descriptive/Core_Competencies_6_07_000.pdf

American College of Nurse-Midwives (ACNM). (2009). *Standards for the practice of midwifery.* Silver Spring: Author. http://www.midwife.org/ siteFiles/descriptive/Standards for Practice_of_Midwifery_12_09_001 .pdf

American Journal of Nursing. (1911). Editorial comments. Room at the top. *12*(2), 85–90. (Available to subscribers only at http://journals.lww.com/ ajnonline/toc/1911/11000)

American Nurses Asssociation (ANA). (2001). *Code of Ethics for Nurses with interpretive statements.* Washington, DC: Nursesbooks.org.

American Nurses Association (ANA). (2007). *ANA principles of environmental health for nursing practice with implementation strategies.* Silver Spring, MD. Nursesbooks.org.

American Nurses Association. (2008). *Professional role competence (Position Statement).* Silver Spring, MD: Author.

American Nurses Association (ANA). (2010). *Nursing's social policy statement: The essence of the profession.* Silver Spring, MD: Nursesbooks.org.

American Nurses Credentialing Center (ANCC). (2008). *A new model for ANCC's Magnet Recognition Program.* Silver Spring, MD: Author.

APRN Joint Dialogue Group. (2008). *The Consensus Model for Advanced Practice Registered Nurses (APRN): Licensure, accreditation, certification and education.* http://www.nursingworld.org/ConsensusModelforAPRN

Benner, P. (1982). From novice to expert. *American Journal of Nursing, 82*(3), 402–407.

Board of Higher Education & Massachusetts Organization of Nurse Executives (BHE/MONE). (2006). *Creativity and connections: Building the framework for the future of nursing education. Report from the Invitational Working Session, March 23-24, 2006.* Burlington, MA: MONE. http://www.mass .edu/currentinit/documents/NursingCreativityAndConnections.pdf

Curtin, L. (2007). The perfect storm: Managed care, aging adults, and a nursing shortage. *Nursing Administration Quarterly, 31*(2), 105–114.

Gallagher-Lepak, S., & Kubsch, S. (2009). Transpersonal caring: A nursing practice guideline. *Holistic Nursing Practice, 23,* 171-182.

Hagerty, B. M. K., Lynch-Sauer, K., Patusky, K. L., & Bouwseman, M. (1993). An emerging theory of human relatedness. *Image, 25,* 291–296.

Institute of Medicine (IOM). (1999). *To err is human: Building a safer health system.* Washington, DC: National Academies Press.

Institute of Medicine (IOM). (2001). *Crossing the quality chasm.* Washington, DC: National Academies Press.

Institute of Medicine (IOM). (2003). *Health professions education: A bridge to quality.* Washington, DC: National Academies Press.

Institute of Medicine (IOM). (2004). *Keeping patients safe: Transforming the work environment of nurses.* Washington, DC: National Academies Press.

Institute of Medicine. (2009). *Forum on the Future of Nursing: Acute care.* "Technology-Enabled Nursing" and "Reactions and Questions" in Chapter 4, Technology, pgs.28-33. Washington, DC: National Academies Press. http://www.nap.edu/catalog.php?record_id=12855

Joynt J. & Kimball, B. (2008). *Blowing open the bottleneck: Designing new approaches to increase nurse education capacity.* Princeton, NJ: Robert Wood Johnson Foundation.

Kane, R.L., Shamilyan, T., Mueller, C., Duval, S. & Wilt, T.J. (2007). *Nurse staffing and quality of patient care.* Rockville, MD: Agency for Healthcare Research and Quality.

Leininger, M. (1988). Leininger's Theory of Nursing: Cultural care diversity and universality. *Nursing Science Quarterly, 1*(4), 152–160.

Appendix A. Nursing: Scope and Standards of Practice, 2nd Edition (2010)

The content in this appendix is not current and is of historical significance only.

National Association of Clinical Nurse Specialists (NACNS). (2008). *Organizing framework and CNS core competencies*. Philadelphia: Author. http://nacns .org/LinkClick.aspx?fileticket=22R8AaNmrUI%3d&tabid=139

National Association of Clinical Nurse Specialists (NACNS). (2009). *Core practice doctorate clinical nurse specialist (CNS) competencies*. Philadelphia: Author. http://www.nacns.org/LinkClick.aspx?fileticket= PAlL7o%2FjOFY%3D&tabid=36

National Organization of Nurse Practitioner Faculties. (2006). *Domains and core competencies of nurse practitioner practice*. Author. http://www .nonpf.com/associations/10789/files/DomainsandCoreComps2006.pdf

Nightingale, F. (1859). *Notes on nursing*. New York: Dover Publications.

Robert Wood Johnson Foundation (RWJF) & Institute of Medicine (IOM). (2009). *Robert Wood Johnson Foundation, Institute of Medicine launch unprecedented initiative on the future of nursing in America*. Princeton, NJ: RWJF. http://www.rwjf.org/pr/product.jsp?id=45714

Stewart, I. M. (1948). *The education of nurses: Historical foundations and modern trends*. New York: Macmillan Company.

Swanson, K. (1993). Empirical development of a middle-range theory of caring. *Nursing Research, 40*(3), 161–166.

Trust for America's Health. (2009). *Making the case: Prevention and health reform*. Washington, DC: Author. http://healthyamericans.org/assets/ files/5.20.09PreventionandReformTPs.pdf

U.S. Department of Health and Human Services (DHHS), Health Resources and Services Administration (2010). The Registered Nurse population: Initial findings from the 2008 National Sample Survey of Registered Nurses. Washington, DC: Author. http://www.bhpr.hrsa.gov/ healthworkforce/msurvey/

U.S. Department of Labor. Bureau of Labor Statistics (2010). *Occupational outlook handbook, 2010–11 edition. Registered nurses*. Washington, DC: Author. http://www.bls.gov/oco/ocos083.htm

Watson, J. (1999). *Postmodern nursing and beyond*. Edinburgh: Churchill Livingstone.

Watson, J. (2008). *Nursing: The philosophy and science of caring*. Boulder, CO: University Press of Colorado.

Appendix B
Nursing's Social Policy Statement: The Essence of the Profession (2010)

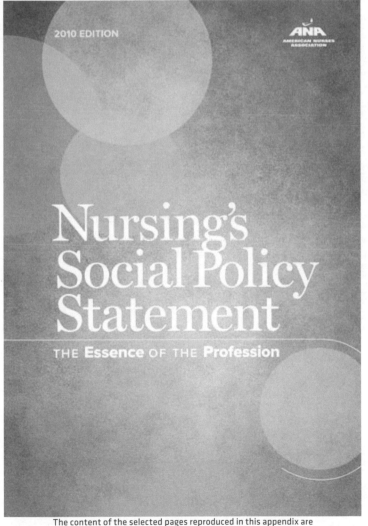

2010 EDITION

ANA
AMERICAN NURSES
ASSOCIATION

Nursing's Social Policy Statement

THE **Essence** OF THE **Profession**

2010 EDITION

Nursing's Social Policy Statement

THE **Essence** OF THE **Profession**

American Nurses Association
Silver Spring, Maryland
2010

Contents

Appendix B. Nursing's Social Policy Statement (2010)

iii

iv   *Nursing's Social Policy Statement*

Appendix B. Nursing's Social Policy Statement (2010)

The content in this appendix is not current and is of historical significance only.

Contributors

Appendix B. Nursing's Social Policy Statement (2010)

Revision of the Social Policy Statement Workgroup, 2009–2010

Catherine E. Neuman, MSN, RN, NEA-BC – Co-Chair
John F. Dixon, MSN, RN, NE-BC – Co-Chair

Bette K. Idemoto, PhD, RN, CCRN, ACNS-BC
Pamela A. Kulbok, DNSc, RN, PHCNS-BC
Jackie R. Pfeifer, MSN, RN, APRN, CCNS
Cheryl-Ann Resha, EdD, MSN, RN
Sue Sendelbach, PhD, RN, CCNS, FAAN
Ann O'Sullivan, MSN, RN, NE-BC, CNE
Kathleen M. White, PhD, RN, CNAA-BC

ANA Staff, 2009–2010

Carol J. Bickford, PhD, RN-BC – Content editor
Katherine C. Brewer, MSN, RN – Content editor
Maureen E. Cones, Esq. – Legal counsel
Yvonne Humes, MSA – Project coordinator
Eric Wurzbacher – Project editor

v

Nursing's Social Policy Statement: An Overview

"Nursing is the pivotal health care profession, highly valued for its specialized knowledge, skill, and caring in improving the health status of the public and ensuring safe, effective, quality care."

(ANA, 2003)

This revision of *Nursing's Social Policy Statement* is the culmination of an extensive review process that also included a long public comment period. It builds on previous editions, especially the original 1980 document. The work describes the essence of the profession by discussing nursing as a profession that is both valued within a society and uniquely accountable to that society. The definition of nursing follows and describes contemporary nursing practice. A more detailed discussion of practice is presented in the sections about the scope and standards of practice and professional performance. A brief commentary about regulation provides an overview of professional, legal, and self-regulation expectations. This foundational ANA publication remains a key resource for nurses both to conceptualize the framework of nursing practice and to provide direction to nursing educators, administrators, and researchers. This publication also can inform other health professionals, legislators and other regulators, those who work in funding bodies, and members of the general public.

1

Social Context
of Nursing

"Nursing is the protection, promotion, and optimization of health and abilities, prevention of illness and injury, alleviation of suffering through the diagnosis and treatment of human response, and advocacy in the care of individuals, families, communities, and populations."

(ANA, 2002)

Nursing, like other professions, is an essential part of the society out of which it grew and within which it continues to evolve. Nursing is responsible to society in the sense that nursing's professional interest must be perceived as serving the interests of society. The mutually beneficial relationship between society and the nursing profession has been expressed as follows:

> Professions acquire recognition and relevance primarily in terms of needs, conditions, and traditions of particular societies and their members. It is societies (and often vested interests within them) that determine, in accord with their different technological and economic levels of development and their socioeconomic, political, and cultural conditions and values, what professional skills and knowledge they most need and desire. By various financial means, institutions will then emerge to train [educate] interested individuals to supply those needs.

> Logically, then, the professions open to individuals of any particular society are the property not of the individual, but of the society. What

3

individuals acquire through training [education] is professional knowledge and skill, not a profession or even part ownership of one. (Page,
1975, p. 7)

The Social Concerns in Health Care and Nursing

Health care continues to be a major focus of attention in the United States and
worldwide. Many other societal concerns garner extensive attention and subsequent action by the nursing profession and its nurse constituency. Nursing
has an active and enduring leadership role in public and political determina-
tions about the following six key areas of health care:

- **Organization, delivery, and financing of quality health care**
  Quality health care is a human right for all (ANA, 2008b). To improve
  the quality of care, healthcare professionals must address these complex
  issues: increasing costs of care; health disparities; and the lack of safe,
  accessible, and available healthcare services and resources.

- **Provision for the public's health**
  Increasing responsibility for basic self-help measures by the individual,
  family, group, community, or population complements the use of health
  promotion, disease prevention, and environmental measures.

- **Expansion of nursing and healthcare knowledge and appropriate
  application of technology**
  Incorporation of research and evidence into practice helps inform the
  selection, implementation, and evaluation processes associated with the
  generation and application of knowledge and technology to healthcare
  outcomes.

- **Expansion of healthcare resources and health policy**
  Expanded facilities and workforce capacity for personal care and community health services are needed to support and enhance the capacity
  for self-help and self-care of individuals, families, groups, communities,
  and populations.

- **Definitive planning for health policy and regulation**
  Collaborative planning is responsive to consumer needs and provides for
  best resource use in the provision of health care for all.

4   *Nursing's Social Policy Statement*

- **Duties under extreme conditions**
  Health professionals will weigh their duty to provide care with obligations to their own health and that of their families during disasters, pandemics, and other extreme emergencies.

Of increasing importance, healthcare regulatory bodies set institutional standards for mandated quality of care, and other healthcare entities provide guidelines and protocols to attain quality care and better outcomes. The goals to provide quality while addressing the costs and quantity of available healthcare services will continue to be social and political priorities for nursing action.

The Authority for Nursing Practice for Nurses

The authority for nursing, as for other professions, is based on social responsibility, which in turn derives from a complex social base and a social contract.

> There is a social contract between society and the profession. Under its terms, society grants the professions authority over functions vital to itself and permits them considerable autonomy in the conduct of their own affairs. In return, the professions are expected to act responsibly, always mindful of the public trust. Self-regulation to assure quality and performance is at the heart of this relationship. It is the authentic hallmark of the mature profession. (Donabedian, 1976)

Nursing's social contract reflects the profession's long-standing core values and ethics, which provide grounding for health care in society. It is easy to overlook this social contract underlying the nursing profession when faced with certain facets of contemporary society, including depersonalization, apathy, disconnectedness, and growing globalization. But upon closer examination, we see that society validates the existence of the profession through licensure, public affirmation, and legal and legislative parameters. Nursing's response is to provide care to all who are in need, regardless of their cultural, social, or economic standing.

The nursing profession fulfills society's need for qualified and appropriately prepared individuals who embrace, and act according to, a strong code of ethics, especially when entrusted with the health care of individuals, families, groups, communities, and populations. The public ranks nurses among the top-few most trusted professionals. In turn, the nursing profession's trusted position in society imposes a responsibility to provide the very best health

Nursing's Social Policy Statement 5

care. The provision of such health care relies on well-educated and clinically astute nurses and a professional association, comprising these same nurses, that establishes a code of ethics, standards of care and practice, educational and practice requirements, and policies that govern the profession.

The American Nurses Association (ANA) is the professional organization that performs an essential function in articulating, maintaining, and strengthening the social contract that exists between nursing and society, upon which the authority to practice nursing is based. That social contract is evident in ANA's most enduring and influential work, which is derived from the collective expertise of its constituent member associations, individual members, and affiliate member organizations. Such work includes:

- Developing and maintaining nursing's code of ethics;
- Developing and maintaining the scope and standards of nursing practice;
- Supporting the development of nursing theory and research to explain observations and guide nursing practice;
- Establishing the educational requirements of professional practice;
- Defining professional role competence; and
- Developing programs and resources to establish and articulate nursing's accountability to society, including practice policy work and governmental advocacy.

The Elements of Nursing's Social Contract

The following statements undergird professional nursing's social contract with society:

- Humans manifest an essential unity of mind, body, and spirit.
- Human experience is contextually and culturally defined.
- Health and illness are human experiences. The presence of illness does not preclude health, nor does optimal health preclude illness.
- The relationship between the nurse and patient occurs within the context of the values and beliefs of the patient and nurse.

6

Nursing's Social Policy Statement

- Public policy and the healthcare delivery system influence the health and well-being of society and professional nursing.

- Individual responsibility and interprofessional involvement are essential.

These values and assumptions apply whether the recipient of professional nursing care is an individual, family, group, community, or population.

Professional Collaboration in Health Care

The nursing profession is particularly focused on establishing effective working relationships and collaborative efforts essential to accomplish its health-oriented mission. Multiple factors combine to intensify the importance of direct human interactions, communication, and professional collaboration: the complexity, size, and culture of the healthcare system and its transitional and dynamic state; increasing public involvement in health policy; and a national focus on health.

Collaboration means true partnership, valuing expertise, power, and respect on all sides and recognizing and accepting separate and combined spheres of activity and responsibility. Collaboration includes mutual safeguarding of the legitimate interests of each party and a commonality of goals that is recognized by all parties. The parties base their relationship upon trust and the recognition that each one's contribution is richer and more truly real because of the strength and uniqueness of the others.

Successful collaboration requires that nursing and its members respond to diversity by recognizing, assessing, and adapting the nature of working relationships with individuals, populations, and other health professionals and health workers. These efforts also extend to relationships within nursing and between nursing and representatives of the public in all environments where nursing practice may occur.

Definition of Nursing

Definitions of nursing have evolved to reflect the essential features of professional nursing:

- Provision of a caring relationship that facilitates health and healing

- Attention to the range of human experiences and responses to health and illness within the physical and social environments

- Integration of assessment data with knowledge gained from an appreciation of the patient or the group

- Application of scientific knowledge to the processes of diagnosis and treatment through the use of judgment and critical thinking

- Advancement of professional nursing knowledge through scholarly inquiry

- Influence on social and public policy to promote social justice

- Assurance of safe, quality, and evidence-based practice

In her *Notes on Nursing: What It Is and What It Is Not*, published in 1859, Florence Nightingale defined nursing as having "charge of the personal health of somebody . . . , and what nursing has to do . . . is to put the patient in the best condition for nature to act upon him."

9

A century later, Virginia Henderson (1961) defined the purpose of nursing as "to assist the individual, sick or well, in the performance of those activities contributing to health or its recovery (or to a peaceful death) that he would perform unaided if he had the necessary strength, will or knowledge. And to do this in such a way as to help him gain independence as rapidly as possible."

In the original *Nursing: A Social Policy Statement* (ANA, 1980), nursing was defined as "the diagnosis and treatment of human responses to actual or potential health problems."

In 2001, ANA's *Code of Ethics With Interpretive Statements* stated that "nursing encompassed the prevention of illness, the alleviation of suffering, and the protection, promotion and restoration of health in the care of individuals, families, groups, and communities."

The definition for nursing remains unchanged from the 2003 edition of *Nursing's Social Policy Statement*:

> Nursing is the protection, promotion, and optimization of health and abilities, prevention of illness and injury, alleviation of suffering through the diagnosis and treatment of human response, and advocacy in the care of individuals, families, communities, and populations.

This definition encompasses four essential characteristics of nursing: human responses or phenomena, theory application, nursing actions or interventions, and outcomes.

Human Responses

These are the responses of individuals to actual or potential health problems, and which are the phenomena of concern to nurses. Human responses include any observable need, concern, condition, event, or fact of interest to nurses that may be the target of evidence-based nursing practice.

Theory Application

In nursing, theory is a set of interrelated concepts, definitions, or propositions used to systematically describe, explain, predict, or control human responses or phenomena of interest to nurses. Understanding theories of nursing and other disciplines precedes, and serves as a basis for, *theory application* through evidence-based nursing actions.

Nursing Actions

The aims of nursing actions (also *nursing interventions*) are to protect, promote, and optimize health; to prevent illness and injury; to alleviate suffering; and to advocate for individuals, families, communities, and populations. Nursing actions are theoretically derived, evidence-based, and require well-developed intellectual competencies.

Outcomes

The purpose of nursing actions is to produce beneficial outcomes in relation to identified human responses. Evaluation of outcomes of nursing actions determines whether the actions have been effective. Findings from nursing research provide rigorous scientific evidence of beneficial outcomes of specific nursing actions.

Figure 1 depicts the intertwined relationships of human responses, theory application, nursing actions, and outcomes.

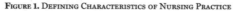

FIGURE 1. DEFINING CHARACTERISTICS OF NURSING PRACTICE

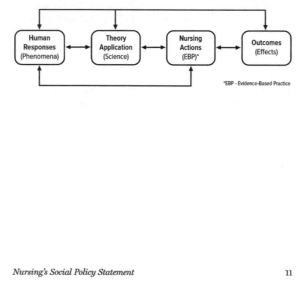

*EBP - Evidence-Based Practice

Appendix B. Nursing's Social Policy Statement (2010)

Knowledge Base for Nursing Practice

Nursing is a profession and is both a science and an art. The knowledge base for professional nursing practice includes nursing science, philosophy, and ethics; biology and psychology; and the social, physical, economic, organizational, and technological sciences. To refine and expand nursing's knowledge base, nurses use theories that fit with professional nursing's values of health and health care and that are relevant to professional nursing practice. Nurses apply research findings and implement the best evidence into their practice based on applicability to the individual, family, group, community, population, or system of care. These efforts generate knowledge and advance nursing science.

Nurses are concerned with human experiences and responses across the life span. Nurses partner with individuals, families, communities, and populations to address issues such as the following:

- Promotion of health and wellness

- Promotion of safety and quality of care

- Care, self-care processes, and care coordination

- Physical, emotional, and spiritual comfort, discomfort, and pain

- Adaptation to physiological and pathophysiological processes

- Emotions related to the experience of birth, growth and development, health, illness, disease, and death

13

- Meanings ascribed to health, illness, and other concepts
- Linguistic and cultural sensitivity
- Health literacy
- Decision making and the ability to make choices
- Relationships, role performance, and change processes within relationships
- Social policies and their effects on health
- Healthcare systems and their relationships to access, cost, and quality of health care
- The environment and the prevention of disease and injury

Nurses use their theoretical and evidence-based knowledge of these human experiences and responses to collaborate with patients and others to assess, diagnose, plan, implement, evaluate care, and identify outcomes. Nursing interventions aim to produce beneficial effects, contribute to quality outcomes, and—above all—do no harm. Nurses use the process that is evidence-based practice as a foundation of quality patient care to evaluate the effectiveness of care in relationship to identified outcomes.

Scope of Nursing Practice

Professional nursing has a single scope of practice that encompasses the range of activities from those of the beginning registered nurse through those of the most advanced level of nursing practice. The scope of practice statement (ANA, 2010) describes the *who, what, where, when, why,* and *how* of nursing practice. Although a single scope of professional nursing practice exists, the depth and breadth to which individual nurses engage in the total scope of professional nursing practice are dependent on their educational preparation and self-development, their experience, their role, the setting, and the nature of the populations they serve.

Further, all nurses are responsible for practicing in accordance with recognized standards of professional nursing practice and the recognized professional code of ethics. Note that the lower level and foundation of the pyramid in Figure 2 *(see next page)* includes the scope of professional practice, standards of practice, and the code of ethics.

Each nurse remains accountable for the quality of care within his or her scope of nursing practice. The level of application of standards varies with the education, experience, and skills of the individual nurse, who must rely on self-determination and self-regulation as the final level of professional accountability.

Professional nursing's scope of practice is dynamic and continually evolving, characterized by a flexible boundary responsive to the changing needs of society and the expanding knowledge base of applicable theoretical and

15

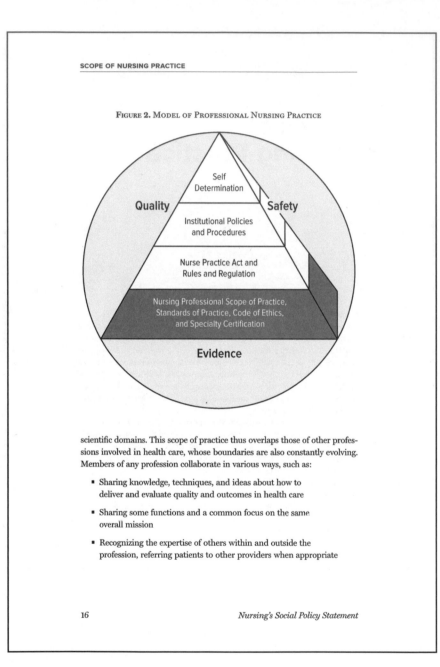

FIGURE 2. MODEL OF PROFESSIONAL NURSING PRACTICE

scientific domains. This scope of practice thus overlaps those of other professions involved in health care, whose boundaries are also constantly evolving. Members of any profession collaborate in various ways, such as:

- Sharing knowledge, techniques, and ideas about how to deliver and evaluate quality and outcomes in health care

- Sharing some functions and a common focus on the same overall mission

- Recognizing the expertise of others within and outside the profession, referring patients to other providers when appropriate

16   *Nursing's Social Policy Statement*

Nursing practice necessitates using such critical-thinking processes as the nursing process to apply the best available evidence to caregiving and promoting human functions and responses. Such caregiving includes, but is not limited to, initiating and maintaining comfort measures, establishing an environment conducive to well-being, providing health counseling, and teaching. Nurses not only independently establish plans of care but also carry out interventions prescribed by other authorized healthcare providers. Therefore, advocacy, communication, collaboration, and coordination are notable characteristics of nursing practice. Nurses base their practice on understanding the human condition across the life span and the relationship of the individual, family, group, community, or population within their own setting and environment.

Registered nurses and nurses with advanced graduate education and preparation provide and direct nursing care. All registered nurses are educated in the art and science of nursing, with the goal of helping individuals, families, groups, communities, and populations to promote, attain, maintain, and restore health or to experience dignified death. Nurses may also develop expertise in a particular specialty. The increasing complexity of care reinforces ANA's consistent advocacy (since 1965) of the baccalaureate degree in nursing as the preferred educational requirement for entry into professional nursing practice.

Specialization in Nursing Practice

Specialization involves focusing on nursing practice in a specific area, identified from within the whole field of professional nursing. ANA and specialty nursing organizations delineate the components of professional nursing practice that are essential for any particular specialty. The following characteristics must be met for ANA recognition of a nursing specialty. A nursing specialty (ANA, 2008d):

- Defines itself as nursing;

- Adheres to the overall licensure requirements of the profession;

- Subscribes to the overall purposes and functions of nursing;

- Is clearly defined;

- Can identify a need and demand for itself;

- Has a well-derived knowledge base particular to the practice of the nursing specialty;

- Is concerned with phenomena of the discipline of nursing;

- Defines competencies for the area of specialty nursing practice;

- Has existing mechanisms for supporting, reviewing, and disseminating research to support its knowledge base;

- Has defined educational criteria for specialty preparation or graduate degree;

- Has continuing education programs or continuing competence mechanisms for nurses in the specialty;

- Is organized and represented by a national or international specialty association or branch of a parent organization;

- Is practiced nationally or internationally; and

- Includes a substantial number of registered nurses who devote most of their practice to the specialty.

Registered nurses may seek certification in a variety of specialized areas of nursing practice as a demonstration of competence (ANA, 2008c).

Advanced Nursing Practice

Advanced nursing practice builds on the competencies of the registered nurse and is characterized by the integration and application of a broad range of theoretical and evidence-based knowledge that occurs as part of graduate nursing education.

Advanced Practice Registered Nurses

Advanced practice registered nurses (APRNs) hold master's or doctoral degrees in nursing, are certified in their designated specialty practice areas, and are recognized and approved to practice in their roles by state boards of nursing or other regulatory oversight bodies, often through special professional licensing processes.

APRNs are educationally prepared in one of the four APRN roles (certified nurse practitioners, certified registered nurse anesthetists, certified nurse-midwives, and clinical nurse specialists) and in at least one of six possible population foci: family/individual across the life span; adult/gerontology; neonatal;

18   *Nursing's Social Policy Statement*

pediatrics; women's health/gender-related health; psychiatric/mental health). Education, certification, and licensure of these individuals should be congruent with role and population foci (APRN Consensus, 2008). APRN specialty practice may focus on specific populations beyond those identified or focus on healthcare needs (such as oncology, palliative care, substance abuse, nephrology) that meet criteria for specialization as identified in the APRN Consensus Model. (See Appendix A for the full text of the APRN Consensus Model.)

Additional Specialized Advanced Nursing Positions

The profession of nursing is also dependent on continued expansion of nursing knowledge, education of nurses, appropriate organization and administration of nursing services, and development and adoption of policies consistent with values and assumptions that underlie the scope of professional nursing practice. Registered nurses may practice in such advanced positions as nurse educator, nurse administrator, nurse researcher, nurse policy analyst, advanced public health nurse, and informatics nurse specialist. These advanced roles require specific additional knowledge and skills gained through graduate level education, holding master's or doctoral degrees.

Further details on the scope of professional nursing practice and the specifics that describe the *who, what, where, when, why,* and *how* of nursing practice for all registered nurses appear in the current version of *Nursing: Scope and Standards of Practice* (ANA, 2010).

Standards of Professional Nursing Practice

To guide professional practice, nursing has established standards of professional nursing practice, which are further categorized into standards of practice and standards of professional performance.

Definition and Function of Standards

Standards are authoritative statements by which the nursing profession describes the responsibilities for which its practitioners are accountable. Standards reflect the values and priorities of the profession and provide direction for professional nursing practice and a framework for the evaluation of this practice. They also define the nursing profession's accountability to the public and the outcomes for which registered nurses are responsible (ANA, 2010).

Development of Standards

A professional nursing organization has a responsibility to its members and to the public it serves to develop standards of practice and standards of professional performance that may pertain to general or specialty practice. The American Nurses Association, as the professional organization for all registered nurses, has assumed the responsibility for developing generic standards that apply to the practice of all professional nurses. However, standards belong to the profession and thus require broad input into their development and

21

revision. The scope and standards of practice developed by ANA describe a competent level of nursing practice and professional performance common to all registered nurses (ANA, 2010).

Standards of Professional Nursing Practice

The Standards of Professional Nursing Practice are comprised of the Standards of Practice and the Standards of Professional Performance.

Standards of Practice

The Standards of Practice describe a competent level of nursing care, as demonstrated by the critical thinking model known as the *nursing process*, which includes the components of assessment, diagnosis, outcomes identification, planning, implementation, and evaluation. These standards encompass significant actions taken by registered nurses and form the foundation of the nurse's decision making.

Standards of Professional Performance

The Standards of Professional Performance describe a competent level of behavior in the professional role, including activities related to quality of practice, education, professional practice evaluation, collegiality, collaboration, ethics, research, resource utilization, and leadership. Registered nurses are accountable for their professional actions to themselves, their patients, their peers, and ultimately to society.

The nursing process is usually conceptualized and presented as the integration of singular, concurrent actions of assessment, diagnosis, identification of outcomes, planning, implementation, and, finally, evaluation. Most often the nursing process is introduced to nursing students as a linear process with a feedback loop from evaluation to assessment, as reflected in Figure 3.

Figure 4 reflects how the nursing process in practice is not linear, but relies heavily on the bidirectional feedback loops from and to each component. The standards of practice are co-located near the steps of the nursing process to represent the directive nature of the standards as the professional nurse completes each component of the nursing process. Similarly, the standards of professional performance relate to how the professional nurse adheres to the standards of practice, completes the nursing process, and addresses other nursing practice issues and concerns.

Appendix B. Nursing's Social Policy Statement (2010)

Appendix B. *Nursing's Social Policy Statement (2010)*

The content in this appendix is not current and is of historical significance only.

FIGURE 3. THE NURSING PROCESS

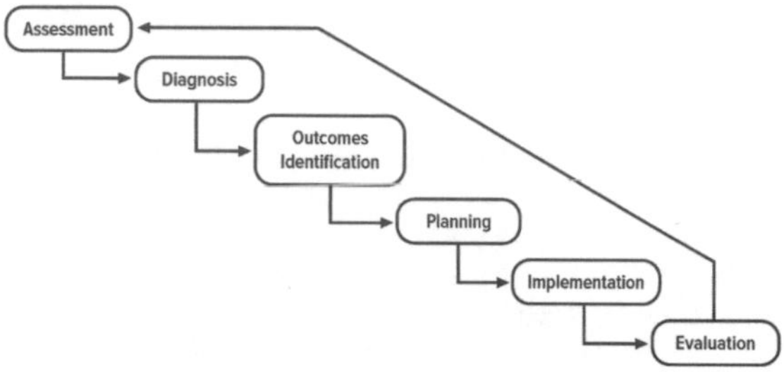

FIGURE 4. THE NURSING PROCESS AND THE STANDARDS
OF PROFESSIONAL NURSING PRACTICE

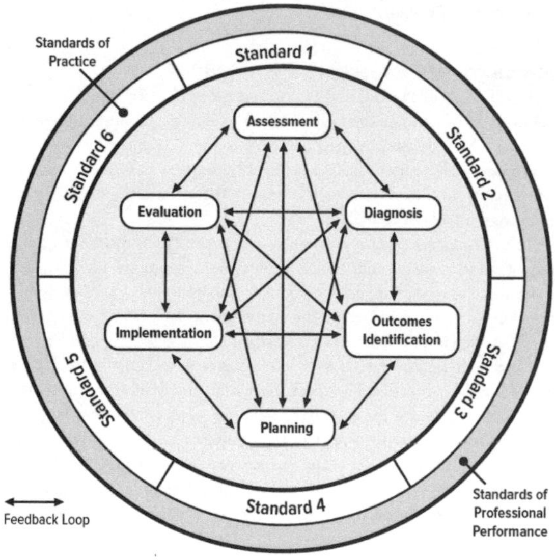

Nursing's Social Policy Statement   23

Application of Scope and Standards

Content within the current edition of *Nursing: Scope and Standards of Practice* should serve as the basis for the following:

- Policies, procedures, and protocols

- Position descriptions and performance appraisals

- Certification activities

- Educational programs and offerings

- Development and evaluation of nursing service delivery systems and organizational structures, including the application of technologies

- Specialty nursing scope and standards of practice

- Quality improvement systems

- Databases

- Regulatory systems

- Healthcare reimbursement and financing methodologies

- Establishing the legal standard of care

Code of Ethics for Nurses

The current code of ethics for the profession, *Code of Ethics for Nurses With Interpretive Statements* (ANA, 2001) "functions as a general guide for the profession's members and as a social contract with the public that it serves" (Fowler, 2008, p. xi). It is the profession's expression of the values, duties, and commitments to that public. Its nine provisions give voice to professional nurses and delineate what the nurse owes not only to others but also to him- or herself. This includes, but is not limited to, personal and professional growth, preserving integrity, and safety (Fowler, 2008).

Although the Code of Ethics for Nurses is intended to be a living document for nurses, and health care is becoming more complex, the basic tenets found within this particular code of ethics remain unchanged. For example, *Guide to the Code of Ethics for Nurses: Interpretation and Application* (Fowler, 2008) provides interpretation and examples of the application of the nine ethical provisions.

Appendix B. Nursing's Social Policy Statement (2010)

Autonomy and Competent Practice

Autonomy is the capacity of a nurse to determine his or her own actions through independent choice within the full scope of nursing practice (Ballou, 1998). Competence is foundational to autonomy: the public has a right to expect nurses to demonstrate professional competence. The nursing profession and professional associations must shape and guide any practice, assuring nursing competence.

The key indicators of competent practice are identified with each standard of practice and professional performance. For a standard to be met, all the listed competencies must be met. An individual who demonstrates competence is performing successfully at an expected level. A *competency* is an expected level of performance that integrates knowledge, skills, abilities, and judgment. Standards should remain stable over time because they reflect the philosophical values of the profession. Competency statements, however, may be revised more frequently to incorporate advances in scientific knowledge and expectations for nursing practice.

Assurance of competence is the shared responsibility of the profession, individual nurses, professional organizations, credentialing and certification entities, regulatory agencies, employers, and other key stakeholders (ANA, 2008c).

The content in this appendix is not current and is of historical significance only.

Appendix B. Nursing's Social Policy Statement (2010)

Regulation of Professional Nursing

Figure 5 *(see next page)* depicts the roles and relationships associated with the regulation of nursing practice. The model recognizes the contributions of professional and specialty nursing organizations, educational institutions, credentialing and accrediting organizations, and regulatory agencies; explains the role of workplace policies and procedures; and confirms the individual nurse's ultimate responsibility and accountability for defining nursing practice (Styles, Schumann, Bickford, & White, 2008).

The Scope of Nursing Practice, the Standards of Professional Nursing Practice, and the Code of Ethics for Nurses serve as the foundation for legislation and regulatory policies to assure protection of the public's safety (Styles, Schumann, Bickford, & White, 2008).

Under the terms of a social contract between society and the profession, society grants authority over functions vital to the profession and permits considerable autonomy in the conduct of its own affairs. Professional nursing, like other professions, is accountable for ensuring that its members act in the public interest while providing the unique service that society has entrusted to them. The processes by which the profession does this include professional regulation, legal regulation, and self-regulation. The Scope of Nursing Practice, the Standards of Professional Nursing Practice, the Code of Ethics for Nurses, and the current social policy statement are components of professional regulation and serve as the foundation for legislation, regulatory policy making, and nursing practice that may be set in place to help assure protection of the public's safety.

27

FIGURE 5. MODEL OF PROFESSIONAL NURSING PRACTICE REGULATION

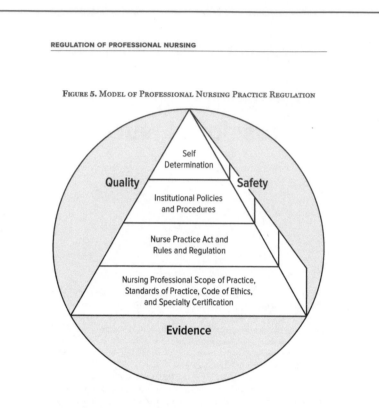

Professional Regulation

Professional regulation is a profession's oversight, monitoring, and control of its members based on principles, guidelines, and rules deemed important. Professional regulation of nursing practice begins with the professional definition of nursing and the delineation of the scope of professional nursing practice. Professional standards are derived from the scope of nursing practice.

The social contract for nursing has been made specific through the professional society's work, derived from the collective expertise of the American Nurses Association, in collaboration with members of its constituent member associations and members of other nursing organizations. These responsibilities include the following:

Appendix B. *Nursing's Social Policy Statement (2010)*

- Establishing and maintaining a professional code of ethics
- Determining standards of practice
- Fostering the development of nursing theory, derived from nursing research
- Establishing nursing practice built on a base of best evidence
- Establishing the specifications for the educational requirements for entry into professional practice at basic and advanced levels
- Developing certification processes as measures of professional competence

Certification is a judgment of competence made by nurses who are themselves practicing within the area of specialization. Certification is the formal recognition of the knowledge, skills, abilities, judgment, and experience demonstrated by the achievement of formal criteria identified by the profession. Credentialing boards develop and implement certification examinations and procedures for nurses who wish to have their specialty-practice knowledge recognized by the profession and the public. One component of the required evidence is successful completion of an examination that tests the knowledge base for the selected area of practice. Other requirements relate to the requisite content of course work and the amount of practice hours. Credentialing bodies may elect to use professional portfolios as psychometrically and legally defensible alternatives for certification examinations. Professional portfolios provide a comprehensive and reflective representation of professional abilities, achievements, and efforts.

Contemporary specialty nursing practice is in transition in response to the increasing complexity of care and exponential explosion of data, information, and knowledge. Specialization is a mark of the advancement of the nursing profession and assists in clarifying, revising, and strengthening existing practice. Specialization not only expedites the production of new knowledge and its application in practice, but also provides preparation for teaching and research related to any defined area of nursing. The specialist in nursing practice is evolving to be a nurse who has become expert in a defined area of knowledge and nursing practice through study and supervised practice at the graduate (master's or doctoral) level.

Legal Regulation

Legal regulation is the oversight, monitoring, and control of designated professionals, based on applicable statutes and regulations, accompanied by the interpretation of these laws. All nurses are legally accountable for actions taken in the course of professional nursing practice, as well as for actions delegated by the nurse to others assisting in provision of nursing care. Such accountability is accomplished through legal regulatory mechanisms of licensure; granting of authority to practice, such as nurse practice acts; and criminal and civil laws.

The legal contract between society and the professions is defined by statute and by associated rules and regulations. State nurse practice acts and related legislation and regulations serve as the explicit codification of the profession's obligation to act in the best interests of society. Nurse practice acts grant nurses the authority to practice and grant society the authority to sanction nurses who violate the norms of the profession or act in a manner that threatens the safety of the public.

Statutory definitions of nursing should be compatible with, and build upon, the profession's definition of its practice base. They must be general enough to provide for the dynamic nature of an evolving scope of nursing practice. Society is best served when consistent definitions of the scope of nursing and of advanced practice nursing are used by each state's board of nursing and other regulatory bodies. This allows residents of all states to access the full range of nursing services. Multiple stakeholders have established a collaborative effort to garner consensus in this arena.

Institutional Policies and Procedures

Nursing practice occurs within societal institutions, organizations, and settings that have accompanying policies, procedures, rules, and regulations. The scope and standards of practice for nursing and nursing specialties should help guide development of institutional policies and procedures to create a more detailed representation of what constitutes safe, quality, and evidence-based nursing practice.

Self-Regulation

Self-regulation, which requires personal accountability for the knowledge base for professional practice, is an individual's demonstrated personal control based on principles, guidelines, and rules deemed important. Nurses develop

30   *Nursing's Social Policy Statement*

FIGURE **6.** Self-Determination in the Model of Professional Nursing Practice Regulation

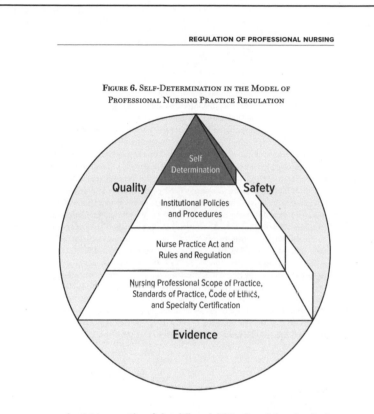

and maintain current knowledge, skills, and abilities through formal academic programs and continuing education professional development programs. When available, nurses pursue certification in their area of practice to demonstrate this competence.

Nurses exercise autonomy and freedom within their scope of practice. Autonomy is defined as the capacity of a nurse to determine his or her own actions through independent choice within the full scope of nursing practice (Ballou, 1998). Autonomy and freedom are based on the nurse's commitment to self-regulation and accountability for practice. In Figure 6, the apex of the pyramid, labeled Self-Determination, represents autonomy, self-regulation, and accountability for practice.

Nursing's Social Policy Statement   31

Competence is foundational to autonomy. Nursing competency is an expected level of performance that integrates knowledge, skills, abilities, and judgment (ANA, 2008d). Greater autonomy and freedom in nursing practice are based on broader authority rooted in expert or advanced knowledge in selected areas of nursing. This expert knowledge is associated with greater self-discipline and responsibility for direct care practice and for advancement of the nursing profession. A greater degree of autonomy not only imposes a greater duty to act and to do so competently but also increases accountability.

Nurses also regulate their own practice by participating in peer review. Continuous performance improvement fosters the refinement of knowledge, skills, and clinical decision-making processes at all levels and in all areas of professional nursing practice. As expressed in the profession's code of ethics, peer review is one mechanism by which nurses are held accountable for practice. As noted in Provision 3.4 (Standards and Review Mechanism) in *Code of Ethics for Nurses with Interpretive Statements*, nurses should also be active participants in the development of policies and review mechanisms designed to promote patient safety, reduce the likelihood of errors, and address both environmental system factors and human factors that present increased risk to patients. In addition, when errors do occur, nurses are expected to follow established guidelines in reporting committed or observed errors. The focus should be directed to improving systems, rather than projecting blame.

Nursing's Social Policy Statement

Application of Nursing's Social Policy Statement

Registered nurses should find the content within *Nursing's Social Policy Statement: The Essence of the Profession* pertinent to everyday practice. The description of nursing as a profession valued within society, definition of nursing, presentation of the nursing process, and discussion of regulation set the stage for practice by promoting understanding.

Nursing faculty should find content within this edition of *Nursing's Social Policy Statement* that is critical for inclusion in curricula and course materials in undergraduate-, graduate-, and doctoral-level education. Similarly, nurses in professional development roles reinforce the concepts presented in this resource in the practice setting, especially those related to autonomy, competence, scope and standards of nursing practice, and the nursing process.

Students will benefit from reading this statement on nursing's social policy as they learn about the evolution of their profession through its key attributes: the definition of nursing, the profession's delineation of the characteristics of a nursing specialty, and the delineation of its scope of practice and accompanying standards and competency statements. The models depicting the nursing process, with its feedback loops and the relationship of the standards of practice and professional performance to the nursing process, will be invaluable in generating improved understanding of the complexity of nursing practice.

33

Appendix B. Nursing's Social Policy Statement (2010)

Similarly, clear delineation of the six social concerns in health care, and other statements that undergird nursing's social contract with society, reaffirm the importance of collaboration within nursing and interprofessional healthcare teams. Registered nurses will experience even greater relevance of this content in every practice setting.

Nurse administrators should use this nursing social policy statement as a resource for strategic planning activities, public explanations about nursing and its registered nurses, and the development of vision and mission statements. Members of legal and regulatory bodies and organizations should review this document to understand better how professional, self-, and legal regulation can complement—rather than conflict with—each other. Healthcare consumers may wish to use the social policy statement to understand better the foundation upon which the nursing profession and its registered nurses base their practice.

Conclusion

This social policy statement describes the pivotal nature and role of professional nursing in society and health care. The definition of nursing, introduction of the scope and accompanying standards of professional nursing practice, and discussion of specialization and regulation within the social context in which nurses practice provide an overview of the essence of nursing. Registered nurses focus their specialized knowledge, skills, and caring on improving the health status of the public and ensuring safe, effective, quality care. This statement serves as a resource to assist nurses in conceptualizing their professional practice and provides direction to educators, administrators, and researchers within nursing. This statement also informs other health professionals, legislators and other regulators, funding bodies, and the public about nursing's social responsibility, accountability, and contribution to health care.

35

References

All web-based references were retrieved May 31, 2010.

American Nurses Association. (1980). *Nursing: A social policy statement.* Kansas City, MO: American Nurses Publishing.

American Nurses Association. (2001). *Code of ethics for nurses with interpretive statements.* Silver Spring, MD: Nursesbooks.org.

American Nurses Association. (2002). *Nursing's agenda for the future: A call to the nation.* http://nursingworld.org/MainMenuCategories/HealthcareandPolicyIssues/Reports.aspx

American Nurses Association. (2003). *Nursing's social policy statement* (2nd ed.). Silver Spring, MD: Nursesbooks.org.

American Nurses Association. (2010). *Nursing: Scope and standards of practice* (2nd ed.). Silver Spring, MD: Nursesbooks.org.

American Nurses Association. (2008a). *Adapting standards of care under extreme conditions: Guidance for professionals during disasters, pandemics, and other extreme emergencies.* Silver Spring, MD: Author.

American Nurses Association. (2008b). *ANA's health system reform agenda.* www.nursingworld.org/healthreformagenda

37

REFERENCES

American Nurses Association. (2008c). *Professional role competence position statement.* http://nursingworld.org/MainMenuCategories/ HealthcareandPolicyIssues/ANAPositionStatements/practice/ PositionStatementProfessionalRoleCompetence.aspx

American Nurses Association. (2008d). *Recognition of a nursing specialty, approval of a specialty nursing scope of practice statement, and acknowledgment of specialty nursing standards of practice.* Silver Spring, MD: Author.

APRN Consensus Work Group & National Council of State Boards of Nursing APRN Advisory Committee. (2008). *Consensus model for APRN regulation: Licensure, accreditation, certification and education.* http:// www.nursingworld.org/ConsensusModelforAPRN

Ballou, K. A. (1998). Concept analysis of autonomy. *Journal of Professional Nursing,* 14(2), 102–110.

Donabedian, A. (1976). Forward, in M. Phaneuf, *The nursing audit: Self-regulation in nursing practice* (2nd ed., p. 8). New York: Appleton-Century-Crofts.

Fowler, Marsha D. M. (Ed.). (2008). *Guide to the code of ethics for nurses: Interpretation and application.* Silver Spring, MD: Nursesbooks.org.

Henderson, V. (1961). *Basic principles of nursing care* (p. 42). London: International Council of Nurses.

Nightingale, F. (1859). *Notes on nursing: What it is and what it is not* (Preface, p. 75). London: Harrison and Sons. (Facsimile ed., J. B. Lippincott Company, 1946).

Page, B. B. (1975). Who owns the profession? *Hastings Center Report, 5* (5, October), 7–8. The Hastings Center: Garrison, NY.

Styles, M. M., Schumann, M. J., Bickford, C. J., & White, K. M. (2008). *Specialization and credentialing in nursing revisited: Understanding the issues, advancing the profession.* Silver Spring, MD: Nursesbooks.org.

Appendix B. Nursing's Social Policy Statement (2010)

Appendix C
ANA Position Statement: *Professional Role Competence* (2014)

On November 12, 2014, the American Nurses Association Board of Directors affirmed the ANA position statement on professional role competency that is produced on the next eight pages, with the following contextual statement:

> The public has a right to expect registered nurses to demonstrate professional competence throughout their careers. ANA believes the registered nurse is individually responsible and accountable for maintaining professional competence. The ANA further believes that it is the nursing profession's responsibility to shape and guide any process for assuring nurse competence. Regulatory agencies define minimal standards for regulation of practice to protect the public. The employer is responsible and accountable to provide an environment conducive to competent practice. Assurance of competence is the shared responsibility of the profession, individual nurses, professional organizations, credentialing and certification entities, regulatory agencies, employers, and other key stakeholders.

Source: http://www.nursingworld.org/MainMenuCategories/Policy-Advocacy/Positions-and-Resolutions/ANAPositionStatements/Position-Statements-Alphabetically/Professional-Role-Competence.html

Position Statements

Professional Role Competence

Effective Date: November 12th, 2014
Status: Affirmed Position Statement
Originated By: Nursing Practice and Work Environment
Adopted By: ANA Board of Directors

Purpose: The purpose of this position statement is to define competence and competency in the professional role of the registered nurse within the context of today's healthcare environment. This position statement also identifies principles for addressing competence in the nursing profession. Initiatives such as the development of the scope and standards of nursing practice, creation of educational curricula, formulation of a research agenda, and revision of the model nurse practice act and other regulatory requirements demand that American Nurses Association (ANA) take a position on this important nursing issue. The work of other professional groups on this topic, i.e. National Council of State Boards of Nursing (NCSBN), nursing specialty groups, and other professional groups, has been reviewed.

Statement of ANA Position: The public has a right to expect registered nurses to demonstrate professional competence throughout their careers. ANA believes the registered nurse is individually responsible and accountable for maintaining professional competence. ANA further believes that it is the nursing profession's responsibility to shape and guide any process for assuring nurse competence. Regulatory agencies define minimal standards for regulation of practice to protect the public. The employer is responsible and accountable to provide an environment conducive to competent practice. Assurance of competence is the shared responsibility of the profession, individual nurses, professional organizations, credentialing and certification entities, regulatory agencies, employers, and other key stakeholders.

© 2014 American Nurses Association

1

ANA believes that in the practice of nursing, competence is definable, measurable and can be evaluated. No single evaluation method or tool can guarantee competence. Competence is situational, dynamic, and is both an outcome and an ongoing process (Competency and Credentialing Institute [CCI], 2008). Context determines what competencies are necessary. The competencies included with each ANA standard of nursing practice are indicators of competent practice for that standard.

History/previous position statements: In May 1999, the ANA Board of Directors appointed an Expert Nursing Panel on Continuing Competence with representation from the State Nurses' Associations (SNA),the ANA board, the American Nurses Foundation (ANF), and the American Academy of Nursing (AAN), the American Nurses Credentialing Center (ANCC), the Nursing Organizations Liaison Forum (NOLF), and the National Council of State Boards of Nursing (NCSBN). This group was charged to develop policy recommendations and an action plan with a proposed research agenda. In August 1999, the ANF board funded a grant titled "The Profession's Action for Continued Competence" to support this work. The ANA Board received the report of the expert panel and authorized review and comments to be sought from the Constituent Member Associations (CMA), the United American Nurses (UAN), the Congress on Nursing Practice and Economics (CNPE), and other related entities (ANA, 2000).

In 2002 the expert panel proposed the Continuing Professional Nursing Competence Process to the ANA House of Delegates. This proposed process incorporated the development of portfolios by individual nurses to document ongoing activities related to the demonstration of continuing competence. The resultant discussion indicated the need for further exploration of this topic.

In 2005 the ANA's Committee on Nursing Practice Standards and Guidelines began a working paper about competence and its relationship to ANA's *Nursing: Scope and*

2

Standards of Practice (ANA, 2004) document. This paper was presented to the Congress on Nursing Practice and Economics (CNPE) in November 2006 for continued development. In May, 2008, the Congress on Nursing Practice and Economics submitted the position statement "Professional Role Competence" to the ANA Board of Directors who subsequently approved the document on May 28, 2008.

Supportive material: ANA's *Nursing's Social Policy Statement: The Essence of the Profession* (2010b) and *Nursing: Scope and Standards of Practice, Second Edition* (2010a) define: "Nursing is the protection, promotion, and optimization of health and abilities, prevention of illness and injury, alleviation of suffering through the diagnosis and treatment of human response, and advocacy in the care of individuals, families, communities, and populations". Therefore, the primary purpose for ensuring competence is the protection of the public. A secondary purpose for ensuring competence is the advancement of the profession through the continued professional development of nurses. A third purpose is to ensure the integrity of professional nursing.

ANA's *Code of Ethics for Nurses with Interpretive Statements* (2001) states: "Individual nurses are accountable for assessing their own competence" (p. 17) and "maintenance of competence and ongoing professional growth involves the control of one's own conduct in a way that is primarily self-regarding. Competence affects one's self-respect, self-esteem, professional status and the meaningfulness of work. In all nursing roles, evaluation of one's own performance, coupled with peer review, is a means by which nursing practice can be held to the highest standards" (p.18). "The nurse owes the same duties to self and to others...to maintain competence, and to continue personal and professional growth" (p. 18).

Definitions and Concepts in Competence

- An individual who demonstrates "competence" is performing successfully at an expected level.
- A "competency" is an expected level of performance that integrates knowledge, skills, abilities, and judgment.
  © 2014 American Nurses Association

3

- The integration of knowledge, skills, abilities, and judgment occurs in formal, informal, and reflective learning experiences.
- Knowledge encompasses thinking; understanding of science, humanities, and professional standards of practice; and insights gained from practical experiences, personal capabilities, and leadership performance.
- Skills include psychomotor, communication, interpersonal, and diagnostic skills.
- Ability is the capacity to act effectively. It requires listening, integrity, knowledge of one's strengths and weaknesses, positive self-regard, emotional intelligence, and openness to feedback.
- Judgment includes critical thinking, problem solving, ethical reasoning, and decision-making.
- Formal learning most often occurs in structured, academic, and professional development environments, while informal learning can be described as experiential insights gained in work, community, home, and other settings.
- Reflective learning represents the recurrent thoughtful personal self-assessment, analysis, and synthesis of strengths and opportunities for improvement. Such insights should lead to the creation of a specific plan for professional development and may become part of one's professional portfolio.

Competence and Competency in Nursing Practice

Competent registered nurses can be influenced by the nature of the situation, which includes consideration of the setting, resources, and the person. Situations can either enhance or detract from the nurse's ability to perform. The registered nurse influences factors that facilitate and enhance competent practice. Similarly the nurse seeks to deal with barriers that constrain competent practice.

The ability to perform at the expected level requires a process of lifelong learning. Registered nurses must continually reassess their competencies and identify needs for additional knowledge, skills, personal growth, and integrative learning experiences.

© 2014 American Nurses Association

4

The expected level of performance reflects variability depending upon context and the selected competence framework or model. Examples of such frameworks for registered nurses include, but are not limited to:

- *Nursing: Scope and Standards of Practice, Second Edition* (ANA, 2010a)
- Specialty nursing scope and standards of practice
- Academic and professional development models (AACN, 2008)
- Benner's Novice to Expert Model (1982)
- Credentialing and privileging requirements
- Statutory and regulatory language
- Evidence-based policy and procedures

ANA's *Nursing: Scope and Standards of Practice, Second Edition* (2010a) is the document defined and promoted by the profession that "describes a competent level of nursing practice and professional performance common to all registered nurses" (p. 2) . Each standard is an "authoritative statement of the duties that all registered nurses, regardless of role, population, or specialty, are expected to perform competently." (ANA, 2010a, p. 2) and "may serve as evidence of the standard of care, with the understanding that application of the standards depends on context (ANA, 2010a, p. 2). Further detailing of the expected level of performance is currently represented as competencies for each nursing process component or professional performance category.

Evaluating Competence

ANA maintains that "…competence can be defined, measured, and evaluated" (ANA, 2010a, p. 12). The competencies included with each standard are key indicators of competent practice for that standard. For a standard of practice or professional performance to be met, all the listed competencies for that standard must be met.

Competence in nursing practice must be evaluated by the individual nurse (self-assessment), nurse peers, and nurses in the roles of supervisor, coach, mentor, or preceptor. In addition, other aspects of nursing performance may be evaluated by professional colleagues and patients/clients.

5

Competence can be evaluated by using tools that capture objective and subjective data about the individual's knowledge base and actual performance and are appropriate for the specific situation and the desired outcome of the competence evaluation. Such tools and methods include but are not limited to: direct observation, patient records, portfolio, demonstrations, skills lab, performance evaluation, peer review, certification, credentialing, privileging, simulation exercises, computer simulated and virtual reality testing, targeted continuing education with outcomes measurement, employer skills validation and practice evaluations. However, no single evaluation tool or method can guarantee competence.

Summary: As the professional association representing the profession of over 3.1 million nurses, ANA leads the profession in addressing the complex issue of assuring professional competence of the nursing workforce.

ANA supports the following principles in regard to competence in the nursing profession:

- Registered nurses are individually responsible and accountable for maintaining competence.
- The public has a right to expect nurses to demonstrate competence throughout their careers.
- Competence is definable, measurable, and can be evaluated.
- Context determines what competencies are necessary.
- Competence is dynamic, and both an outcome and an ongoing process.
- The nursing profession and professional organizations must shape and guide any process assuring nurse competence.
- The competencies contained in ANA's various scope and standards of practice documents are the competence statements for each standard of nursing practice and of professional performance.
- Regulatory bodies define minimal standards for regulation of practice to protect the public.
- Employers are responsible and accountable to provide an environment

6

conducive to competent practice.

- Assurance of competence is the shared responsibility of the profession, individual nurses, regulatory bodies, employers, and other key stakeholders.

Recommendations/Next Steps

The definitions of competence and competency and the accompanying descriptions of related concepts were incorporated in ANA's *Nursing: Scope and Standards of Practice, 2nd Edition* (2010a).

Many issues and questions remain and must be addressed, including but not limited to:

- How does the work environment impact the assurance and maintenance of competence?
- How should basic competence or specialized competence be measured?
- Who pays for it?
- What are the legal issues related to the assurance and maintenance of competence?
- How will or should competency measurement be used in licensure and regulation? (Whittaker, Carson, & Smolenski, 2000)
- What are the implications of competence for nurses who practice as part of interprofessional teams?

ANA affirms its commitment to ongoing examination, discussion, and action related to these and other issues around competence of nurses.

References

American Association of Colleges of Nursing. (2008). *The Essentials of Baccalaureate Education for Professional Nursing Practice*. Retrieved October 18th 2014 from http://www.aacn.nche.edu/education-resources/BaccEssentials08.pdf

American Nurses Association. (2000). *Continuing competence: Nursing's agenda for the*

7

21st century. Washington, DC: American Nurses Association

American Nurses Association. (2001). *Code of ethics for nurses with interpretive statements.* Washington, DC: nursebooks.org.

American Nurses Association. (2004). *Nursing: Scope and standards of practice.* Silver Spring, MD: Nursesbooks.org.

American Nurses Association. (2010a). *Nursing: Scope and standards of practice, second* edition. Silver Spring, MD: Nursebooks.org.

American Nurses Association. (2010b). *Nursing's social policy statement..* Silver Spring: MD: Nursebooks.org.

Benner, P. (1982). From novice to expert. *American Journal of Nursing.* 82(3), 402-407.

Competency and Credentialing Institute (CCI). (2008). *The CCI continued competence leadership forum: From pieces to policy post-event white paper.* Retrieved October 18th, 2014 from http://www.cc-institute.org/docs/default-document-library/2011/10/19/fromPiecesToPolicy.pdf?Status=Master

Whittaker, S., Carson, W., & Smolenski, M. (2000). Assuring continued competence-policy questions and approaches: How should the profession respond? *Online Journal of Issues in Nursing,* Retrieved October 20th, 2014 from http://nursingworld.org/MainMenuCategories/ANAMarketplace/ANAPeriodicals/OJIN/TableofContents/Volume52000/No3Sept00/ArticlePreviousTopic/ContinuedCompetence.html.

8

Appendix C. ANA Position Statement: Professional Role Competence (2014)

Appendix D
The Development of Essential Nursing Documents and Professional Nursing

The American Nurses Association has long been instrumental in the development of three essential documents for professional nursing: its code of ethics, its scope and standards of practice, and its statement of social policy. Each document contributes to further understanding the context of nursing practice at the time of publication and reflects the history of the evolution of the nursing profession in the United States.

Advancing communication technologies have expanded the revision process to permit ever-increasing numbers of registered nurses to contribute to the open dialogue and review activities. This ensures that the final published versions not only codify the consensus of the profession at the time of publication, but also reflect the experiences of those working in the profession at all levels and in all settings.

A Timeline of Development

1859   Florence Nightingale publishes *Notes on Nursing: What It Is and What It Is Not.*

1896   The Nurses' Associated Alumnae of the United States and Canada is founded. Later to become the American Nurses Association (ANA), its first purpose is to establish and maintain a code of ethics.

1940   A "Tentative Code" is published in *The American Journal of Nursing,* although never formally adopted.

1950   *Code for Professional Nurses,* in the form of 17 provisions that are a substantive revision of the "Tentative Code" of 1940, is unanimously accepted by the ANA House of Delegates.

1952   *Nursing Research* publishes its premiere issue.

1956   *Code for Professional Nurses* is amended.

1960   *Code for Professional Nurses* is revised.

1968   *Code for Professional Nurses* is substantively revised, condensing the 17 provisions of the 1960 Code into 10 provisions.

1973   ANA publishes its first *Standards of Nursing Practice.*

1976   ANA publishes *Standards of Gerontological Nursing Practice*, its first such publication for a nursing specialty practice.

1976   The *Code of Ethics for Nurses with Interpretive Statements,* a modification of the provisions and interpretive statements, is published as eleven provisions.

1980   ANA publishes *Nursing: A Social Policy Statement.*

1985   The National Institutes of Health organizes the National Center for Nursing Research.

        ANA publishes *Titling for Licensure.*

        The *Code of Ethics for Nurses with Interpretive Statements* retains the provisions of the 1976 version and includes revised interpretive statements.

        The ANA House of Delegates forms a task force to formally document the scope of practice for nursing.

1987   ANA publishes *The Scope of Nursing Practice.*

1990   The ANA House of Delegates forms a task force to revise the 1973 *Standards of Nursing Practice.*

1991   ANA publishes *Standards of Clinical Nursing Practice.*

1995   ANA publishes *Nursing's Social Policy Statement.*

1995   The Congress of Nursing Practice directs the Committee on Nursing Practice Standards and Guidelines to establish a process for periodic review and revision of nursing standards.

1996   ANA publishes *Scope and Standards of Advanced Practice Registered Nursing.*

1998   ANA publishes *Standards of Clinical Nursing Practice, 2nd Edition* (also known as the *Clinical Standards*).

2001   The *Code of Ethics for Nurses with Interpretive Statements,* a modification of the eleven 1976 provisions and the 1985 interpretive statements, is accepted as nine provisions by the ANA House of Delegates in July and published in September.

        ANA publishes *Bill of Rights for Registered Nurses.*

2002   ANA publishes *Nursing's Agenda for the Future: A Call to the Nation.*

2003   ANA publishes *Nursing's Social Policy Statement, 2nd Edition.*

2004   ANA publishes *Nursing: Scope and Standards of Practice.*

2008   The APRN Consensus Model is published by the APRN Consensus Work Group and APRN Joint Dialogue Group.

ANA publishes *Professional Role Competence Position Statement.*

ANA publishes *Specialization and Credentialing in Nursing Revisited: Understanding the Issues, Advancing the Profession.*

2010   ANA publishes *Nursing's Social Policy Statement: The Essence of the Profession.*

ANA publishes *Nursing: Scope and Standards of Practice, 2nd Edition.*

2014   The *Code of Ethics for Nurses with Interpretive Statements*, a modification of the nine provisions and their interpretive statements of 2001, is approved by the ANA Board of Directors (November).

2015   ANA publishes *Code of Ethics for Nurses with Interpretive Statements.*

ANA publishes *Nursing: Scope and Standards of Practice, 3rd Edition.*

Appendix E
Selected Nurse Theorists

Theorist	Model/Theory
Anne Boykin & Savina Schoenhofer	Nursing as Caring Theory
Barbara Dossey	Theory of Integral Nursing
Joanne Duffy	Quality Caring Model
Helen Erickson, Evelyn Tomlin & Mary Ann Swains	Modeling and Role Modeling
Dorothy Johnson	Behavioral System Model
Imogene King	Theory of Goal Attainment
Katherine Kolcaba	Comfort Theory
Madeleine Leininger	Theory of Culture Care Diversity and Universality
Myra Levine	Conservation Model
Rozzano Locsin	Technological Competency as Caring and the Practice of Knowing Persons in Nursing
Merle H. Mishel	Uncertainty in Illness Theory
Betty Neuman	Neuman Systems Model
Margaret Newman	Health as Expanding Consciousness
Florence Nightingale	Environmental Model of Nursing
Ida Jean Orlando (Pelletier)	Nursing Process Theory
Dorothy Orem	Self-Care Deficit Theory
Rosemary Rizzo Parse	Humanbecoming School of Thought
Josephine Paterson & Loretta Zderad	Humanistic Nursing Theory
Hildegard Peplau	Theory of Interpersonal Relations

(continued)

Theorist	Model/Theory
Marilyn Ann Ray	Theory of Bureaucratic Caring
Pamela Reed	Theory of Self-Transcendence
Martha E. Rogers	Science of Unitary Human Beings
Sister Callista Roy	Roy Adaptation Model
Marlaine Smith	Theory of Unitary Caring
Mary Jane Smith & Patricia Liehr	Story Theory
Kristen Swanson	Theory of Caring
Jean Watson	Theory of Human Caring and Caring Science

Appendix F
Culturally Congruent Practice Resources

Diversity and Cultural Competency Resources

American Association of Colleges in Nursing: Cultural Competency in Nursing Education
http://www.aacn.nche.edu/education-resources/cultural-competency

Transcultural Nursing Standards of Practice

http://www.tcns.org/TCNStandardsofPractice.html

Specialty Nursing Organizations and Related Groups

American Assembly of Men in Nursing
http://aamn.org

Asian American/Pacific Islander Nurses Association
http://www.aapina.org

Association of Black Nursing Faculty
http://www.abnf.net

Health Professions for Diversity Coalition
http://www.hpd-coalition.org

National Alaska Native American Indian Nurses Association
http://www.nanainanurses.org

National American Arab Nurses Association
https://n-aana.org/Index.asp

National Association of Hispanic Nurses
http://www.thehispanicnurses.org

National Black Nurses Association
http://www.nbna.org

National Coalition of Ethnic Minority Nursing Associations (NCEMNA)
http://www.ncemna.org

Philippine Nurses Association of America
http://www.philippinenursesaa.org

Sullivan Alliance to Transform America's Health Profession
http://www.jointcenter.org/new_site/sullivan.htm

Bibliography for Additional Sources on Culturally Congruent Care

Common search terms to use on sites below include *health disparities, cultural competence, CLAS standards, racial* and *ethnic disparities,* and *diversity.*

Agency for Healthcare Research and Quality (2014). National Healthcare Quality & Disparities Report, pp. 8–10
http://www.ahrq.gov/research/findings/nhqrdr/nhqdr14/index.html

American Association of Colleges of Nursing
www.aacn.nche.edu/qsen/workshop-details/.../KD-PCC-Toolkit.pdf

Association of American Colleges and Universities
http://www.aacu.org/american_commitments/curr_fac_dev_network.cfm

American Association of Medical Colleges. "Tools for Assessing Cultural Competence Training"
https://www.aamc.org/initiatives/tacct/

American Hospital Association
http://www.aha.org/search?q=cultural+competence&site=redesign_aha_org|HPOE

Assessment tools for cultural competency
http://www.transculturalcare.net

Center for Cross-Cultural Health
http://www.crosshealth.com/ccch/whatwedo.html
http://www.crosshealth.com/ccch/publications.html

Center for Disease Control (CDC) Prevention Research Center Program
http://www.cdc.gov/prc/about-prc-program/index.htm

Center for Human Diversity
http://www.centerforhumandiversity.org/

Cross Cultural Health Care Program
http://xculture.org

Cultural Case Studies. Fanlight Productions
http://www.fanlight.com/catalog/films/912_wa.php

DiversityRX
http://diversityrx.org

Health Sciences Library (Search for *cultural competence*)
http://libweb.lib.buffalo.edu/
(Highlights resources that help nursing faculty and other interested professionals incorporate cultural competence skills into nursing curricula and practice.)

Institute of Medicine (IOM). Report on Racial & Ethnic Disparities
https://www.iom.edu/Reports/2002/Unequal-Treatment-Confronting-Racial-and-Ethnic-Disparities-in-Health-Care.aspx

International Council of Nurses (ICN)
http://icn.ch/index.html

The Joint Commission (Search for *CLAS standards*, *cultural competence*)
www.jointcommission.org

The Joint Commission International
www.jointcommissioninternational.org

Kaiser Permanente (Search for *diversity programs*, *language services*, etc.)
http://www.kaiserpermanente.org

Mayo Clinic, Office of Diversity
http://www.mayoclinic.org

National Center for Cultural Competence. Georgetown University
http://www.georgetown.edu

National Center on Minority Health and Health Disparities (NCMHD)
www.ncmhd.nih.gov/

National Coalition of Ethnic Minority Nurse Associations (NCEMNA)
www.ncemna.org

National Consortium for Multicultural Education for Health Professionals
http://culturalmeded.stanford.edu/teaching/publications.html
http://culturalmeded.stanford.edu/teaching/culturalcompetency.html

National Institute of Health (NIH) (Search for *health disparities*)
http://www.nih.gov

National Institute of Minority Health. (U.S. Department of Health and Human Services)
http://www.nih.gov/about/almanac/organization/NIMHD.htm

National Library of Medicine (PubMed, Medline Plus, etc.)
http://nlm.nih.gov

National Quality Form. National Quality Forum (NQF)
http://www.qualityforum.org

Healthcare disparities and cultural competency
http://www.qualityforum.org/projects/Healthcare_Disparities_and_
Cultural_Competency.aspx#t=2&s=&p=

RAND Health: Survey Tools
http://www.rand.org/health/surveys_tools.html

The California Endowment
www.calendow.org

Principles and Recommended Standards for Cultural Competence
Education of Health Care Professionals
http://www.diversityrx.org/resources/principles-and-recommended-
standards-cultural-competence-education-health-care-professiona

Think Cultural Health
http://www.thinkculturalhealth.hhs.gov

Transcultural Nursing Society. Links to transcultural nursing theories and
models
http://www.tcns.org

United Nations (UN)
www.un.org

United States Agency for International Development (USAID)
http://www.usaid.gov

U.S. Department of Health and Human Services, Agency for Healthcare
Research and Quality
http://www.ahrq/gov/

U.S. Department of Health and Human Services, Health Resources and
Services Administration (HRSA). Culture, Language and Health Literacy
http://www.hrsa.gov/culturalcompetence/index.html

U.S. Department of Health and Human Services. Office of Disease
Prevention and Health Promotion. *Healthy People 2020*, November 2010
http://www.healthypeople.gov/2020/about/DisparitiesAbout.aspx

U.S. Department of Health and Human Services, Office of Minority Health
http://minorityhealth.hhs.gov

U.S. Department of Health and Human Services. Center for Linguistic and Cultural Competency in Health Care
http://minorityhealth.hhs.gov/omh/browse.aspx?lvl=2&lvlid=34

U.S. Department of Health and Human Services. National Standards for Culturally and Linguistically Appropriate Services (CLAS)
http://minorityhealth.hhs.gov/omh/browse.aspx?lvl=2&lvlid=53

World Health Organization (WHO). (Search for *cultural competency, health disparities*)
http://who.int

Index

Note: Entries designated with [2010] indicates content from *Nursing: Scope and Standards of Practice*, 2nd Edition. That information is not current, and is of historical value only.

A

acculturation, definition of 85

advanced practice registered nurses (APRNs)
- advanced practice competencies involving 56
- advanced practice roles 42, 42–43
- APRN Consensus Model 38
- certified nurse midwives (CNMs) 42
- certified nurse practitioners (CNPs) 42
- certified registered nurse anesthetists (CRNAs) 42
- clinical nurse specialists (CNSs) 42
- competencies involving 54, 56, 60, 62, 64, 65, 66, 70, 72, 73, 75, 77, 80, 83, 84
- definition of 2, 85
- educational programs for 42–43
- licensure, accreditation, certification, and education (LACE) 42
- roles of [2010] 125–126
- types of 2–3

advocacy 33
- definition of 20
- individual level 20
- interpersonal level 20
- nursing practice and 20
- organization and community level 20
- policy level 20

Affordable Care Act 30

Agency for Healthcare Research and Quality (AHRQ) 28

American Association of Critical-Care Nurses 26–27

American Holistic Nurses Association (AHNA) 26

American Journal of Nursing 17, 38

American Nurses Association (ANA) 1, 22, 23, 35, 213, 223
- developing scope and standards 1
- essential nursing documents, development timeline of 223–226
- position statement on competence 213–222
- support for professional competencies 45

American Nurses Credentialing Center (ANCC) 24
- The Magnet Recognition Program 24

American Nurses Credentialing
Center (continued)
    Pathway to Excellence
        Program 25
Andrews/Boyle Transcultural
    Interprofessional Practice Model
    (TIP) 31
ASKED (Awareness, Skill,
    Knowledge, Encounters,
    Desire) 32
assessment
    competencies involving 53–54,
        54, 56, 57, 60
    definition of 85
    parameters 53
    Standards of Practice 4, 53–54
    Standards of Practice
        [2010] 139–140
assessment data, competencies
    involving 55, 66
autonomy, definition of 85

B

baby boomers 48–49
Bureau of Labor Statistics (BLS) 39
    employment projections 46

C

care coordination 9, 28–29. *See
    also* coordination of care
caregiver, definition of 85
care giving. *See also* nursing care
    cultural components of 13
    definition of 11, 12
    interventions and 12
    nursing practice and 7–8, 11–12
    team-based 28
    theory and science of 12
    transcultural literacy and 13
care studies 17

caring, definition of 85
    holistic 88
Certified Nurse Midwives (CNMs) 2,
    3, 40, 42
Certified Nurse Practitioners
    (CNPs) 3, 42
Certified Registered Nurse
    Anesthetists (CRNAs) 2, 3, 40,
    42
Clinical Nurse Specialists (CNSs) 3,
    42
clinical research 17. *See also* nursing
    research
*Code of Ethics for Nurses with
    Interpretive Statements* xi, 10, 22,
    35, 36–37, 67, 81, 86, 224, 225
    competencies for 35
    provisions of 36–37
code of ethics (nursing), definition
    of 86
collaboration
    competencies involving 57, 61,
        62, 63, 65, 66, 68, 73, 74,
        78, 79
    definition of 86
    interprofessional 9
    Standards of Professional
        Performance and 5, 73–74
    Standards of Professional
        Performance and
        [2010] 164–165
communication
    competencies involving 53, 55,
        61, 62, 65, 69, 71, 74, 75, 84
    Standards of Professional
        Performance and 5, 71–72
    Standards of Professional
        Performance and [2010] 161
competence in nursing practice
    ANA position statement
        on 213–221
    evaluation of 45

competencies for nursing
practice 9–10, 43–45, 49–50.
See also competencies for nursing
standards
evidence-based 18, 18–19
range of needed by nursing
students 47
competencies for nursing
standards 6, 51. *See
also* advanced practice
registered nurses; graduate-level
prepared registered nurses; *See
also* competencies for nursing
practice; *See also* each standard in
Standards of Practice; Standards
of Professional Performance
advanced practice registered
nurses (APRNs) 54, 56, 60,
62, 64, 65, 66, 70, 72, 73,
75, 77, 80, 83, 84
assessment 53, 54, 56, 57, 60,
66
assessment data 55
collaboration 57, 61, 62, 63, 65,
66, 68, 73, 74, 78, 79
communication 53, 55, 61, 62,
65, 69, 71, 74, 75, 84
coordination of care 57, 63
cultural components of care 53,
54, 55, 57, 58, 61, 62, 65,
68, 71, 79
cultural issues 57
data and information in nursing
practice 55, 61, 64, 66, 67,
79, 80
diagnosis 54, 55, 57, 59, 60, 66,
80
education 69, 70, 73, 76
environmental health 84
ethics 54, 57, 58, 62, 77, 78, 81
evaluation 57, 65, 66, 70, 78,
79, 80, 82
evidence-based practice and
research 54, 57, 59, 60, 61,
65, 70, 77, 79, 80

expected outcomes 55, 57
graduate-level prepared registered
nurses 54, 55, 57, 60, 61, 63,
65, 66, 70, 72, 73, 75, 77,
79, 80, 82, 84
health teaching and health
promotion 65
implementation 61
leadership 75
outcomes identification 57
planning 55, 59, 61, 63, 65, 66,
70, 73, 74, 79
prescriptive authority 62
professional practice
evaluation 81
quality issues 57, 62, 65, 68, 73,
74, 75, 77, 82
quality of practice 79
resource utilization 82
self-care in nursing practice 63, 68
self-evaluation 81
self-reflection 68, 76, 81
tests and procedures 54
competency, definition of 44, 86
*Consensus Model for APRN
Regulation: Licensure,
Accreditation, Certification, and
Education* 42
consultation and Standards of
Practice and [2010] 150
continuity of care, definition of 86
continuous quality improvement 9
coordination of care. *See also* care
coordination
competencies involving 57, 63
Standards of Practice and 4,
63–64
Standards of Practice and
[2010] 147
*Core Competencies for Basic Midwifery
Practice* 42
*Core Practice Doctorate Clinical Nurse
Specialist (CNS) Competencies* 43
credentialing 41

ethical characteristics of the
professional nurse 36
ethical conduct of research and
nursing practice 10
ethics
competencies involving 54, 57,
58, 62, 67, 77, 78, 81
Standards of Professional
Performance and 5, 67–68
Standards of Professional
Performance and
[2010] 154–155
evaluation. *See also* profesional
practice evaluation
competencies involving 57, 65,
66, 70, 78, 79, 80, 82
data and 66
definition of 87
expected outcomes and 87
Standards of Practice and 5, 66
Standards of Practice and
[2010] 152–153
evidence-based competencies
cost measures and 18
outcome measurement and 18
evidence-based practice and
research. *See also* nursing
research; clinical research
competencies involving 54, 57,
59, 60, 61, 65, 70, 77, 79, 80
Standards of Professional
Performance and 77–78
Standards of Professional
Performance and [2010] 158
evidence-based practice (EBP) 9,
17, 18. *See also* evidence-based
practice and research
definition of 87
framework for 18–19
Standard of Professional
Performance and 6
translational research and 19–20
evidence-based practice (EBP)
[2010] 122–124

expected outcomes 57
competencies involving 55, 57
definition of 87
diagnosis and 86
evaluation and 87
outcomes identification and 57
planning and 89

F

family, definition of 87
fatigue and nursing 22–23
Federation of State Medical
Boards 28
*Forming, Storming, Norming,
Performing Model* 28
The Future of Nursing 30
Future of Nursing Campaign 30

G

Giger & Davidhizar's Transcultural
Assessment Model 32
graduate-level prepared registered
nurses
competencies involving 54, 55,
57, 60, 61, 63, 65, 66, 70,
72, 73, 75, 77, 79, 80, 82, 84
definition of 2, 87

H

healing 11
health
definition of 87
nursing practice and 7–8
social determinants of 30
health care 31
expectations of millennial
generation 48
pressure to cut expenses
of 48–49
reformation of 45
team-based improvement
of 29–31

healthcare consumer-centered approach 9

healthcare consumer-centered practice 9

healthcare consumers 2, 8
    definition of 2, 88

healthcare home 46

healthcare professionals, core compentencies of 9–10

healthcare providers, definition of 88

healthcare services, framework for change in 29

health teaching and health promotion
    competencies involving 65
    Standards of Practice and 4, 65

The HEALTH Traditions Model 32

Healthy Nurse
    constructs 23–24
        authority to advocate 24
        calling to care 24
        opportunity to role model 24
        priority to self-care 24
        responsibility to educate 24
    framework 23–24

Healthy People 2020 30, 49, 53
    assessment parameters 53

healthy work environments 21
    American Association of Critical-Care Nurses 26
    American Nurses Association (ANA) and 23–24
    appropriate staffing 26
    authentic leadership 26
    constructs for 23–24
    core values and 26
    effective decision-making 26
    factors influencing 21
    healthy nurse framework 23–24
    meaningful recognition 26
    optimal domains for 27–28
    optimal staffing for 23–24
    Pathway to Excellence Program 25
    Safe Patient Handling and Mobility (SPHM) 22
    Samueli Institute 27
    skilled communication in 26
    standards for establishing and maintaining 26–27
    supports for 23–27
    true collaboration and 26

heath teaching and health promotion
    Standards of Practice [2010] 148–149
    Standards of Practice and [2010] 148–149

Henry Street Settlement House 38

holistic approach 11–12, 16
    core values of 26
    nursing process and 9

holistic care, definition of 88

Holistic Nursing: Scope and Standards of Practice 26

hotspotting 49–50

human caring. *See* care giving

Human Caring Science Theory 11

I

illness, definition of 88

implementation
    competencies involving 61
    holistic definition of 88
    planning of 61–62
    Standards of Practice and 4, 61–62
    Standards of Practice and [2010] 145–146

incivility. *See* workplace violence

individualization of nursing practice 8

informatics 9

information, definition of 88

Institute of Medicine (IOM) 28
    nurse participation in 30
interdisciplinary education 47–48
interprofessional
    collaboration 9
        definition of 88
    collaborative practice domains 27
    competency, definition of 27
    definition of 88
    education 47
    teams 27–28, 32, 46
interventions 12

J

Jeffreys's Cultural Competence and
    Confidence (CCC) Model 32

K

*Keeping Patients Safe: Transforming the
    Work Environment of Nurses* 29
knowledge translation
    cost analysis and 19
    plans 19
    synonyms of 19

L

leadership
    competencies involving 75
    Standards of Professional
        Performance and 5, 75
    Standards of Professional
        Performance and
        [2010] 162–163
licensure. *See* registered nurses
    (RNs), licensure of
licensure, accreditation, certification,
    and education (LACE) 42

M

The Magnet Recognition
    Program 24

empirical outcomes 25
exemplary professional
    practice 24
model components of 24–25
new knowledge, innovation, and
    improvements 24
structural empowerment 24
transformational leadership 24
Massachusetts Institute of
    Technology (MIT) 28
Medicaid Expansion 30
medical home 46
millennial generation, health care
    expectations of 48
Model of Professional Nursing
    Practice Regulation 33–36
models
    Andrews/Boyle Transcultural
        Interprofessional Practice
        Model (TIP) 31
    Culture Care Diversity and
        Universality 31
    Giger & Davidhizar's Transcultural
        Assessment Model 32
    The HEALTH Traditions
        Model 32
    Jeffreys's Cultural Competence and
        Confidence (CCC) 32
    The Process of Cultural
        Competence in the Delivery of
        Health Services 31
    professional nursing practice
        regulation 33–36
    Purnell Model for Cultural
        Competence 32

N

National Academy of Sciences 29
National Association of Boards of
    Pharmacy 28
National Center for Nursing
    Research 17

National Council Licensure
Examination for Registered
Nurses (NCLEX-RN) 41
National Council of State Boards of
Nursing 28, 35, 39
National Institute for Occupational
Safety and Health (NIOSH) 22
National Institutes of Health 17
National Sample Survey of
Registered Nurses 39
Nightingale, Florance 17, 35, 96
    epidemiologic models influenced
        by 18
nurse
    attorneys 21
    leaders 29
    theorists 17, 227–228
nurse practice acts 35, 36, 61
nurse practitioners (NPs) 40
nursing. *See also* nursing practice
    advanced titles for 38
    advocacy 7, 20, 33
    art of 11–12
    art of [2010] 130
    care coordination and 9
    care studies and 17
    caring relationships 12
    clinical research and 17
    commitment to the profession
        [2010] 133
    creating a sustainable
        workforce 46–47
    credentialing 41
    culturally congruent practice 31
    definition of 1, 7, 49, 88
    definition of [2010] 108
    demand for 40
    development of essential nursing
        documents 223–226
    education 30, 38
    employment projections for 40,
        46–47
    ethical characteristics of 36

evidence-based practice (EBP) 17,
    18, 19–20
external influences on 31
fatigue and 22–23
focuses 7
holistic approach
        actions of 16
        transcultural literacy
            and 13
the how of 9
inclusion of "facilitation of healing"
    and "groups" 1
integrating science and art of 6–7
integrating science and art of
    [2010] 129–130
interprofessional collaboration
    and 9
objectives 31
optimal staffing and 23–24
organizations 229–230
outcome measures and 19
patients and 11
practice areas 39–40
professional education
    requirements for 37
professional practice
    boundaries 32–33
prospectively 16
responsibilities to society 10
retrospective circumstances
    and 16–17
roles in reformed and restructured
    care delivery system 46–47
safe work environment and 22
science of 13
science of [2010] 129
social contract with society 10
societal and ethical dimensions of
    [2010] 131
specialization 37–38, 38–39
specialty practice in
    [2010] 124–125
teams 28–30
technology advances and 48
theorists 227–228

nursing (continued)
    theory 17, 36
    timing for 16–17
    traditional strengths of 28–29
    transcultural standards of
        practice 229
    trends and issues
        [2010] 133–136
    ways of knowing and 17
    when it occurs 16–17
    workplace violence and 22
Nursing: A Social Policy
    Statement 10. *See also* Nursing's
    Social Policy Statement
nursing care and registered nurses
    (RNs) 33–34
nursing education 17–19, 47–48.
    See also education
    continuous learning 41
    credentialing 41
    curricula design 47
    specialization 41
nursing education [2010] 127
nursing knowledge 17
    development of 17
Nursing Outcomes Classification 19
nursing practice
    advocacy and 7, 20
    and caring [2010] 132–133
    caring and health 7–8, 11–12
    and the Code of Ethics for
        Nurses 10
    compentancy in all healthcare
        settings 49–50
    competence in [2010] 119–120
    competencies
        data and information 53
        interprofessional 27–28
        professional 43–44
    critical thinking and 6–7
    culturally congruent 9, 31
    data and information
        competencies and 55, 61, 64,
        66, 67, 79, 80

    definition of 2–3, 88
    description of 2–3
    description of [2010] 109
    development and function of 3–4
    environments for 19–21
    epidemiologic models and 18
    ethical conduct of research
        and 10
    evidence-based 9, 13, 17
        competencies 18–19
        knowledge 17
    evidence-based practice (EBP) 18
    evidence-based practice (EBP)
        [2010] 122–124
    healthcare consumer-centered
        approach 9
    healthcare consumers and 8
    healthy work environments 21
    healthy work environments
        [2010] 112, 112–114
    holistic consumer-centered care 7
    individualization of 8
    manner of 10
    methods of 9–10
        situation, background,
            assessment,
            recommendation
            (SBAR) 9–10
        TeamSTEPPS 9–10
    model of professional nursing
        practice regulation of 33–36
        policies and procudures
            for 35
        rules and regulations
            governing 35
        scope and standards
            of practice, code of
            ethics, and specialty
            certification 35
        self-determination in 35
    nursing knowledge, development
        of 17
    optimal health outcomes 7
    research and 19–20
    science of 6–7

patient care, team-based approach
to 29
peer review, definition of 89
plan, definition of 89
planning
    competencies involving 55, 59,
      61, 63, 65, 66, 70, 73, 74, 79
    expected outcomes and 89
    implementation of 61–62
    outcomes identification and 57
    Standards of Practice and 4,
      59–60
    Standards of Practice and
      [2010] 143–144
*Population-focused Nurse Practitioner
  Competencies* 43
prescriptive authority
    competencies involving 62
    Standards of Practice and
      [2010] 151
Principles for Nurse Staffing 23
The Process of Cultural Competence
  in the Delivery of Health Services,
  Model 31
professional code of ethics. *See
  also* Code of Ethics for Nurses
    registered nurses (RNs) and 33
professional licensure. *See* registered
  nurses (RNs), licensure of
professional competence in nursing
  practice. *See* competence in
  nursing practice
professional nursing. *See* nursing
professional nursing practice.
  See nursing practice
professional practice evaluation
    competencies involving 81
    Standards of Professional
      Performance and 6, 81
    Standards of Professional
      Performance and [2010] 166
Professional Role Competence
  (2014) 213–222

Purnell Model for Cultural
  Competence 32

Q

quality
    competencies involving 57
    continuous improvement and 9
    definition of 89
quality issues, competencies and 62,
  65, 68, 73, 74, 75, 77, 82
Quality of Health Care in America
  Committee 29
quality of life 11, 31, 63
quality of practice
    competencies involving 79
    Standards of Professional
      Performance and 6, 79–80
    Standards of Professional
      Performance and
      [2010] 159–160

R

registered nurses (RNs) 3
    advocacy and 20
    care coordination and 9
    and the Code of Ethics for
      Nurses 10
    core compentencies of
      practice 9–10
    credentialing 41
    critical thinking and 6–7
    culturally congruent practice 9
    definition of 2, 89
    determination of the total
      supply 39
    education and 32
    evidence-based practice 9
    graduate-level prepared, definition
      of 87
    graduate-level prepared
      competencies and 54, 55, 57,
      60, 61, 63, 65, 66, 70, 72,
      73, 75, 77, 80, 82, 84

registered nurses (continued)
    healthcare consumer-centered
      approach 9
    interprofessional collaboration
      and 9
    interprofessional teams 32
    knowledge translation and 19
    licensure, accreditation,
      certification, and education
      (LACE) 42
    licensure of 41–42
      requirements 41
    manner of practice 10
    nursing care and 33–34
    professional code of ethics and 33
    professional competencies
      for 43–44
    projected job openings for 46–47
research. *See* nursing research;
  clinical research; evidence-based
  practice and research
resource utilization
    competencies involving 82
    Standards of Professional
      Performance and 6, 82–83
    Standards of Professional
      Performance and [2010] 167
retrospective circumstances 16–17
Robert Wood Johnson Foundation
  (RWJF) 28

S

*Safe Patient Handling and Mobility
  Interprofessional National
  Standards* 22
safe patient handling and mobility
  (SPHM) 22
Samueli Institute 27
Scope of Nurse Anesthesia Practice 42
Scope of Nursing Practice 1, 3
    definition of 2–3, 89
    description of 2–3
    development and function of 3–4

tenents of nursing practice
  and 7–9
self-care in nursing practice 24, 27
  competencies involving 63, 68
self-determination 35, 36
self-evaluation, competencies
  involving 81
self-reflection, competencies
  involving 76, 81
self-reflection 27
  competencies involving 68
situation, background, assessment,
  recommendation (SBAR) 9–10
social accountable care
  organization 49–50
social contract 10
social determinants of health 30
specialty practice in nursing 37–38
  credentialing of 41
specialty practice in nursing
  [2010] 124–125
staffing issues in nursing practice. *See
  also* optimal staffing
*Standards for Accreditation of
  Nurse Anesthesia Educational
  Programs* 43
*Standards for Nurse Anesthesia
  Practice* 42
*Standards for the Practice of
  Midwifery* 43
Standards of Practice 1, 4–5, 13,
  15, 26, 35, 42, 49, 53, 81
    assessment 4, 6, 53–56
    assessment [2010] 139–140
    competent level of nursing practice
      and 15
    consultation [2010] 150
    coordination of care 4, 63–64
    coordination of care [2010] 147
    definition of 89
    diagnosis 4, 55–56
    diagnosis [2010] 141

W

Wald, Lillian 37
wellness, definition of 89
WHO (World Health
    Organization) 53
        assessment parameters 53

work environments and
    technology 48. *See also* healthy
    work environments
workplace violence 22
work teams. *See* teams
worldview, definition of 89